"After you read this book you will never be the same. Through scientific research translated with passion into laypersons language you will have enough information to not only question authority, but do something about it. Wait until you read these facts! You will be astonished at where we are <u>letting</u> our leaders take us and our children. This book will teach you about your rights, be afraid no more, you can stand up for yourself and your family."

—Julia A. Trebing, Psy.D Stamford, Connecticut

"I absolutely LOVE this book! Finally, someone is just telling it like it is. You get to the truth quickly on every page without having to read through a ton of B.S. first. Dr. Trebing, I salute you and your brave efforts. Your book is all about helping children, families and the planet."

—Dr. Robert Egy, Naturopathic Physician, Boulder CO.

"This book has given me all the intelligent ammunition I have needed to keep my kids safe from the medical Gestapo. We are no longer afraid!

—R. Montrose, Boston MA (father of 2)

"I did not believe a word of this until I heard Dr. Trebing speak in our small church in Houston. Now I am on a crusade and my entire family, including all my nieces and nephews, are clean of medical vermin. Over the two years we have switched to no shots, cleaner diets and no medicines they have never been healthier. My son's 10 year trauma with asthma is gone! You really need to read and incorporate this book into your life."

—Tamara Williams, Houston Texas (mother or 4)

"I was getting violently sick from the flu shots my employer made me get every year at the hospital I give massages at. I used some of the forms in this book and they backed off immediately. I have not had a flu shot in 2 years and I have been far healthier and happier."

—Dawn Ruben, massage therapist Los Angeles

"I went through hell with the school districts and the DCF here in Baltimore. They were trying to get my kids vaccinated regardless of my beliefs, and threatened to put them in foster homes. I went to work with the help of this book and God's grace. I attacked them back for 2 months with these forms, and I could not believe how the tide changed! They became apologetic, started blaming each other, and in the end after several negotiations all my kids are in the public schools here in Baltimore without shots! Part of the agreement was that I be quiet and never tell anyone, and I thought this was what I needed to do since I had been through so much. But I am now thinking of writing my own book about the experience! Dr. Trebing, bless you for saving my family from these demons."

—L. Jefferson, Baltimore MD (mother of 6)

"I have two daughters, one has chronic asthma and allergies and the other became autistic a few weeks after vaccines were given. The doctors office denied any correlation to the shots, but I knew they were lying. I began feeding them better and organic foods, got them totally off dairy, and of course stopped giving them shots after my first reading of Good-Bye Germ Theory. I think I was one of the first people to buy the first edition. My first daughter now has no asthma, and my second is coming out of her autism with therapeutic listening therapy. I home school now to avoid persecution and to protect my children."

—Lois Reed, NYC (mother of 3)

"While I have investigated many alternative modalities and concepts with a high degree of skepticism, I found Dr. Trebings' book to be well founded in fact and scientific evidence on the impact that vaccination can have on your health. Good-Bye germ theory is a radically different paradigm that represents common sense which today, unfortunately, is not prevalent in our culture, school systems or government. This book is an easy read that anyone can use to gain knowledge about making responsible health choices for themselves or their family, coupled with the ammunition to assert your rights in making these choices. I highly recommend this book to all my patients!"

—Ken Barrett, DC Sacramento California

GOOD-BYE
GERM THEORY

GOOD-BYE GERM THEORY

Ending A Century Of Medical Fraud and How to Protect Your Family

Dr. William P. Trebing

To order additional copies of this book, contact:
Xlibris Corporation
1-888-795-4274
www.Xlibris.com
Orders@Xlibris.com
24660

CONTENTS

For suffering children all the world over

Disclaimer

Dr. William P. Trebing is not a lawyer, and does not claim, imply or suggest to be in any way, nor is it the intent of this book to give legal advice. Nor do any of the people involved in MD publishing, who have graciously printed and published this text. The information contained herein has been researched as much as possible to insure accuracy. However unlikely, there are no claims being made here that there are no errors. You are encouraged to go to your own local law library and department of public records to examine the related documents for yourself, or acquire the services of a licensed lawyer or law student to certify their validity. *The information dispensed within this book IS NOT for the purpose of providing legal advice.* It is for educational purposes only. What you do with it after that is totally your choice and responsibility.

Understand there is always a risk involved when you stand up for your rights within the confines of a corrupted judicial system that does not support them. There is a lot of power, money and political influence purporting the fraud in which this text is attempting to expose. Therefore, if you use the information in this book and in updates thereto to help yourself and your family, you do so at your own risk. The authors and publishers disclaim any responsibility or liability for any use and application, either directly or indirectly, of any information from this book or updates. The book was written for informational and educational purposes only, from a non-licensed, layman research perspective with concern to anything within that may be construed as "legal advice." This text is not an offer for anything in commerce.

Respectively, the author accepts the Oaths of Office of any and all Officials in the Public who may obtain and read this text.

To order more books

Fill out the form below and send $25
($20 for the book and $5 S&H) to:
MD Publishing House
34 Arcadia Road, #683
Old Greenwich, CT 06870
Allow 2 weeks for delivery
You may call (203) 661-8122 to arrange a book
order pick up @ $20 per book
Or you may order on line at
www.xlibris.com/goodbyegermtheory.html
www.amazon.com
www.barnesandnoble.com
www.borders.com

Book Order Form

For
Good-Bye Germ Theory

Name _____ Address _____

State _____ Zip _____ Phone _____

When you need a quick fact
in a hurry!

✓ Autism has increased by over 3,000 times since the advent
   of mandatory vaccination programs, when it was considered
   very rare. The medical profession blames this on new
   diagnostic parameters, but this alone could not possibly
   have created such a drastic increase in so little time. The
   systematic blood poisoning of America's children through
   mercury and other products in vaccines is the only event
   which could possibly do this.

✓ Following mandatory vaccine programs one of every 149
   children in Brick Township, NJ is Autistic. Following
   mandatory vaccine programs between 1993 and 1998,
   Autism increased 513% in the state of Maryland.

✓ Doctors are instructed by the American Medical Association
   to "downplay" parents concerns of vaccine reactions, and
   to deny any correlation of adverse reaction to vaccines they
   have just administered.

✓ Federal government reports confirm that vaccinations kill
   more than 3 children per week in America.

✓ Jonas Salk, national hero and creator of the famous "Salk"
   polio vaccine made a public statement in 1976 that two
   thirds of the cases of polio which occurred between 1966
   and 1976 were caused by his vaccine.

✓ The DPT shot has been banned in most of Europe and
   Japan since 1975 due to it's extreme toxicity, but American
   children still receive this vaccine.

✓ Records prove that the death rates from polio, pertussis,
   whooping cough and measles were decreasing on their own

before the vaccine was introduced, and that present records were altered to demonstrate the decrease was due to vaccines.

✓ Each year, there are approximately 950 deaths from the whooping cough vaccine, as compared to 10 deaths from the actual disease.

✓ Drug companies use the same pertussis shot to intentionally create encephalitis in experimental lab animals.

✓ Over 95% of people who actually acquire diseases have been vaccinated against those very diseases. Drug companies refuse to study unvaccinated populations.

✓ The *"Germ Theory"* does not follow any scientific guideline to prove its' validity. When assessed by the simple *"scientific method"* taught in elementary schools, it is proven invalid.

✓ Pasteur's major credits did not belong to him, but to another brilliant scientist called Pierre Bechamp, who totally disagreed with Pasteur's *"germ theory"* of disease creation. Most of Pasteur's early vaccine work ended in disaster.

✓ Early studies demonstrate how all bacteria, fungi and virus all originate from the same parent organism, which is a natural healthy component to all living things.

✓ The Center for Disease Control charters an Epidemic Intelligence Service, which travels the country in search of symptoms they can use to formulate epidemics for profit.

✓ Forcefully vaccinating anyone can be considered assault and battery.

✓ Most vaccination laws are completely unconstitutional, and have no relevance to today's world. Local Health Departments promote most vaccination programs to acquire Federal Aid and Grant money at the expense of America's children.

✓ Everyone who wishes can enter a courtroom *Pro Se,* or *Sui Juris,* without the high cost of a lawyer, and WIN! You do not have to be vaccinated, or have your children vaccinated against your will. Taking the proper time with important sovereignty foundation paperwork, filed with your town clerks office, can also help protect you and your family, while avoiding courts, judges and lawyers all together.

✓ The FDA has reported that doctors under-report vaccine reactions by 90%.

✓ In any given population, the majority of people who become ill are those who are vaccinated.

✓ Unvaccinated populations can be proven scientifically and otherwise far healthier than vaccinated ones.

✓ Encephalitis (brain damage due to swelling of brain tissue) is an almost given side effect to vaccine toxins according to most research studies on vaccine damages.

✓ 15 to 20% of American school children are considered to be learning disabled with brain damage dysfunction directly caused by vaccines.

✓ Your government pays out tens of thousands of tax dollars each year to cover vaccination damage claims.

✓ Unvaccinated populations are far healthier than vaccinated ones', however no medical or government organization wishes to study them.

✓ Your child is 94 times more likely to die from a whooping cough vaccine than from the actual whooping cough, and nearly 4,000 times more likely of acquiring long-term damage from the vaccine than from developing the disease.

✓ The CDC is aware that Thimerosal (mercury preservative in vaccines) is linked to Autism by virtue of their own private research. However they refuse to provide the raw data from these studies, as requested by congressman Dan Burton (R-Indiana), to be used for an independent review by a third party research organization.

✓ Giving a ten-pound infant a single vaccine in a day is the equivalent of giving a 100 pound adult 40 vaccines in a day.

✓ Considering the above information, medical doctors insist on injecting 45 vaccines directly into your child's blood stream by age 6 months; 64 by age 18 months; and 74 by age 6.

✓ The CDC has an Advisory Committee on Immunization Practices, called the ACIP. This committee advises lawmakers as to which vaccines should be mandated. The

ACIP is riddled with conflicts of interest, since committee members own patents for vaccines and stock in the pharmaceutical companies which make the vaccines.

✓ Americans are amongst the most vaccinated people in the history of the planet, and are also amongst the sickest in it's history. Half of all Americans suffer with at least one chronic disease, and one fifth have 2 or more. These chronic diseases cause 70% of all American deaths.

How to educate your pediatrician

The majority (certainly not all) of the pediatricians you meet have huge egos supported by an over developed sense of importance and self righteousness. They believe their limited knowledge is enough to dictate control of your child, through either medical or police state measures. Most, as well, are people just like you and I who can be reached, and enlightened by the facts. If your pediatrician can not give you satisfactory answers to your concerns about vaccines, or worse yet, refuses to, it's high time to search for one who will. You should go over every fact on the previous pages' *"Fact in a hurry"* sheet with your pediatrician. The chart which follows will also be of help in your query. If your pediatrician has made a statement not mentioned below, please send it to us at the address located on page 2, and we will follow up with an answer based in fact and science.

If your pediatrician says   *Then answer*

"Vaccines are completely safe."   *Ans.#1 "then why does the packet insert to each one list dozens of possible side effects, including death?"*
                                       Ans.#2 "Since you're so sure, will you please put that in writing?"
                                       Ans. #3 "These vaccines contain mercury, which Is a scientifically proven neurotoxin, as well as aluminum and formaldehyde. How can you assure that these poisons won't hurt my child?"

"People and books which challenge vaccines believe flawed research."

"Research which warns the people of the dangers of vaccines has been completed by competent and respected doctors in all professions from many Universities in America and abroad. Most hold medical or microbiology degrees. Also, much of the positive research on vaccines can be considered flawed by denying standing facts, and from being conducted by the very companies which create the vaccines."

Ans #2 : "Can you cite a specific study which assures the safety of the vaccines you want to administer?

"Not vaccinating your children is an irresponsible and dangerous parenting chioce."

"Choosing to not vaccinate is anything but irresponsible. The choice requires a lot of research, and is certainly more responsible than blindly following medical advice in light of ever growing reports of neurological damage to children created by vaccines."

"If you do not vaccinate your child you are violating the law. You can be arrested and your child can be taken away from you."

Ans.#1 "You are not a lawyer. Please do not preach to me the law, since I have already researched it."

Ans.#2 "Neither myself nor my child can be forcefully medicated, against my will. If these vaccines are mandated by law, then the law, and you as a doctor must also assure me that my child will not be harmed by these mandated vaccines in any way. Further, I want to be assured that these mandated vaccines are going to prevent the very diseases they are given for. Sign these papers assuring me of just that and I will vaccinate."

"If you do not vaccinate your child is at risk of developing some serious disease that can kill them!"

"If vaccines truly work, as you believe they do, and if the bulk of our society's children are vaccinated, than my child should have nothing to worry about. Unless of course you really don't believe that vaccines work."

"They can still get the disease from a child who carries the germ, or from the environment!"

"You are contradicting yourself doctor. If vaccines truly work then there should be no carrier children. Secondly, there is no proof that these so called germs you speak of are lurking around in the environment waiting to attack my child. We live under very sanitary conditions. Thirdly, in any given population it has been shown that kids who get sick have already been vaccinated. The bulk of unvaccinated children do not get sick."

"Vaccines wiped out polio in the 50's"

"Considering that the creator of the polio vaccine, Jonas Salk, reported that two thirds of polio cases between '66 and '76 were created by his vaccine, you are making a huge assumption there doctor. Fact is, that polio naturally began to decline around '53, and the vaccine wasn't promoted until '57. After the vaccine to this very day, spinal meningitis, a disease which is virtually identical to polio, has been present in epidemic proportions."

"Vaccines have ended many childhood diseases like measles and mumps. Kids are less sick today because of vaccines."

"In any given population children still get sick with the very diseases vaccines are reported to have ended. Studies show that more than 95% of these sick children have already been vaccinated for the disease they now have."

"People are living longer today for two main reasons; vaccines and antibiotics."

"Autism and vaccines have no relation, proven by valid medical research."

"Medical research proves that more autism is reported today not due to vaccine damage, but due to vast changes in the diagnosis of the disorder. Before the changes only a few characteristics were associated with autism. Now there are many."

"Medicine likes to take credit for people living longer, however nothing can be further from the truth. Antibiotics have helped people who are in trouble with certain infections, however research shows that chronic antibiotic use leads to more sickness and disease. Many studies show that disease and vaccine data have been altered by the pharmaceutical companies to show a favorable result for vaccines use. Without this trickery they could not promote their programs through government."

"Doctors always say this without really knowing what they are talking about. Autism occurs quite often after a child has come home from receiving a dose of vaccines. Vaccines contain toxins like mercury that have been proven to cause brain damage, sudden infant death syndrome and cancer in children."

"No single change in diagnostic parameters for any disease has ever caused it to increase more than 3,000% in 15 years, as is the case with autism. Only one thing can create such a drastic increase so quickly, and that is the systematic neurological poisoning of a population created by neuro-toxins found in vaccines."

"Antibody tests are the "TELL ALL" for the Diagnosis of any given disease where immunity is Involved. Antibodies are produced in the presence of germs, which proves that germs cause disease."

"That is rhetorical nonsense doctor. Antibody tests for the determination of any one disease have been proven up to 75 % inaccurate. Every manufacturer of antibody tests shows at least a 35% margin of error. People with high antibody levels get sick every day, while those with low antibody levels appear to be immune. There are many levels to immunity; antibodies are just one level and may not be a reliable indication of immunity. Show me some real science!"

"The new chicken pox vaccine is a major break through in modern medicine and greatly reduce your childs' chances of getting the disease."

"The chicken pox vaccine has been tested will minimally, and then only by the drug company who creates it. Children who take Homeopathic remedies for chicken pox can get through the process in 36 hours. Studies have been completed by independent researchers showing that 95% of vaccinated children still get chicken pox. Other studies show that chicken pox may be a step in the natural development of the child's immune system.

Foreward

If we were to evaluate many of the practices we take for granted in society, we'd be in for quite a surprise. Scratch below the surface of much of what is "accepted," and you'll discover a most amazing world, a world of intense debate where scientific studies can and often do arrive at conflicting and often opposite conclusions; differing philosophies clash, valid yet unpopular research and ideas are ignored or suppressed, while bad ideas are promoted. You may see hidden agendas, conflicts of interest and power struggles. Are we talking about some freakish state of affairs?

Sadly, the answer is no. From Flower Club meetings, to the PTA, from corporations, research laboratories and medical journals to the halls of Congress we often see politicking, rumor-milling, selfishness, distrust and backstabbing. We may also see brilliance, insight, genius, honor, civility, trust, caring, altruism and honesty.

This state of affairs is given a special name; its called human nature.

One may wonder how people can accomplish anything, and yet our civilization's achievements have reached to the heavens, literally and figuratively.

It has not been an entirely uphill climb, we've often fallen back.

While vacationing in London recently my family and I visited the Theatre Museum of the National Museum of the performing arts. Our guide led us through a hallway filled with dioramas depicting the history of the theatre in England. The first model was of an early theatre.

"This theatre, built in the 1600s was the first theatre in England since Roman times."

Imagine that. In the fifth century the Roman legions left England to defend a crumbling empire from the threatening barbarian hordes. They never returned. The ravaging Vandals, Goths, Huns, Saxons, Celts and others enslaved people, destroyed homes, books, libraries, works of art, temples, churches, schools and other cultural institutions that the classical civilizations of Greece and Rome took over a thousand years to create. It was dissolved amidst chaos to be replaced by a thousand years of Dark Ages.

For over a thousand years, no theatres were built.

Human progress has not been an unbroken line moving upwards and onwards. We have fallen back. We can always fall back.

We like to mouth platitudes such as "truth will prevail" but it often does not. Without eternal vigilance civilization can crumble. The barbarians are never far from our gates. It was not too long ago that the world was nearly drowned in the barbarism of Fascism and Communism. What is the next "ism" to threaten our freedoms? How can we best recognize it?

History shows us that a people with just laws based on tolerance and respect for individual freedoms and property can create a free, strong society that can defend it's borders, engage in trade, educate its young and promote the general welfare. Such are the best protections against barbarism.

But when conflicts of interest and selfishness predominate we get intolerance, bad laws, innumerable edicts (regulations), confiscatory taxation, poor education, a powerful bureaucracy before which the people cringe, and a corrupt, overbearing government which creates a distrust of our institutions and decay of our culture. "When the people are strong the government is weak and when the government is strong the people are weak" is a wise Chinese saying.

Rome, and nearly every great civilization has fallen more from within than from without; the rot had been spreading long before the enemy arrived at the gates. The Romans themselves had lost their ideals and had become barbarians in their own way.

The barbarians threaten us today. Yet today's barbarians are not wild looking hairy conquerors lurking just outside our borders, ready to sack our cities, carry citizens off into slavery and burden us with heavy tribute.

Today's barbarians live amongst us, dress like us and use our language. Yet they poison our minds with junk science and damage our society with unconstitutional laws. They are a meddling bureaucracy, which includes government officials who believe they can and should, regulate any area of our lives they wish. They are private agencies and special interest groups who push for laws and regulations to control others. They have forgotten the ideals of separation of power, rule of law, the sacredness of one's being, property and personal beliefs—the ideals upon which civil society rest.

Many of today's barbarians are the product of a school system whose purpose is to create conforming and socialization rather than inspire learning, creativity and education. How could a state employed teacher, certified by the state, using state approved texts, teaching state approved subjects, following a state approved syllabus teach students to become independent thinking citizens to question the status quo? These teachers are the product of the same "educational" system. Barbarians teaching our children to become barbarians.

Perhaps barbarian is not the right word. These are weak people we're creating—followers who go along to get along and do not know how to think for themselves, question and speak up.

Are we educating children who will one day lead us and recreate government, education and society to preserve our life, liberties and freedoms so the pursuit of happiness may flourish? Or are we creating a generation that will passively
   watch the freedoms that were so valiantly fought for slip away in front of their TVs?

The rot is from within. As Pogo said: "We have met the enemy and they is us."

What can we do? We must educate our children and ourselves to see below the thin veneer of the "accepted ways", to the conflicting science, philosophies and ideals that helped create and re-create our civilization. To touch the inspiration from which our ideals derive, to understand our roots.

·Without periodically dipping into that well-spring of thought our world will become stagnant and the rot will spread; our children will not understand the philosophies and struggles that brought us to our present state of life, freedom and liberty. They will not be able to recognize threats to our life, freedom and liberty.

As we explore our roots, we may discover that some of the generally accepted ways of doing things exist because of political power and the stifling of debate, and they should be changed. We will surely discover that many of yesterday's norms must continue to be cherished and protected.

In this text, *Good-bye Germ Theory*, Dr. William P. Trebing looks beneath the veneer and investigates areas of human endeavor that have become stagnant, dogmatic and suppressive of dissent, such as medicine and law.

Dr. Trebing asks us to look at the unconscious ways we have been thinking and acting, and to engage in a healthy questioning and reevaluation of the accepted premises upon which these areas of our lives are based.

Tedd Koren, DC Jan 3rd, 2002. Gwynedd Valley, PA
Founder of Koren Publications. Visit us online
www.korenpublications.com

Prologue

Welcome to a life transforming experience! Good-bye Germ Theory: Ending a Century of Medical Fraud.

Finally a book, like no other book. A book that tells all. There's no mincing of words here. If you are searching for the truth, search no more. This grass roots effort is gaining momentum and attention. Get on board, get educated, give your children that extra chance, be the Hundredth Monkey* that tunes into an awareness, strengthens the field and pushes our society's consciousness energy where Dr. Trebing knows we must go.

After you read this book you will never be the same. Through scientific research translated with passion into laypersons language you will have enough information to not only question authority, but do something about it. Wait until you read these facts! You will be astonished at where we are *letting* our leaders take us and our children. This book will teach you about your rights, be afraid no more, you can stand up for yourself and your family.

Dr. Trebing, a scientist by nature, is a deeply committed physician, husband and father. He is smart, honest, sassy, and has an uncommon love for all children. All this weaved together with him being a richly, spiritual man results in his truth containing a light that no darkness can diminish.

Inspired on many levels, but driven to write this book after Autism came to his neighborhood, this information is a compilation of Dr. William P. Trebing's brilliant life's work. A no fear, forthright style that puts the truth out there undeniably. This stuff is scary, uncomfortable, but to be empowered, for change to happen, we all need to know it and respond to protect our families! We need this man to stand up for us and our children, until we can do it ourselves. He is a welcome departure from those other advocates that stand on the fence, too ignorant or afraid to speak the whole truth. He is a leader for our times, willing to say it like it is, with all the facts to back him up. He assesses the problems and tells you the solutions. He kicked me so hard off that fence that I was on the ground digging with him and running to educate others all at the same time.

I wondered out loud, 'Why it is easier for most physicians to medicate so many people rather than to get just one of them to change their lifestyle?' Dr. Trebing simply says, "Never give up!" I greatly respect and love the way this man thinks.

Toni Morrison said "the function of freedom is to free someone else. Welcome to freedom thanks to Dr. William P. Trebing.

Sleep well,
Dr. Julia A. Trebing
Director of Creative Therapies
Stamford Connecticut
Psychological Services for Children & Families

Introduction

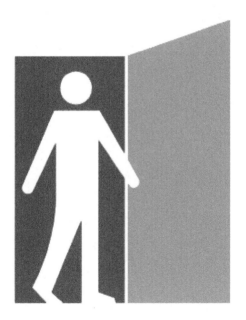

For those of you familiar with the movie, *"The Matrix,"* you have a very clear choice here and now to either take the blue or the red pill. Take the blue pill, and you stop right now, go back to reading your New York Times, taking medications, receiving vaccinations, believing everything you are told by your medical doctor, eventually becoming sick and dying of some disease like 90% of the human beings walking the Earth today. Take the red pill, and like Morpheus, I show you how deep the rabbit hole goes. The choice is yours. One caveat; embarking on the pages of this book should be carefully considered by worshipers of Big Brother and the faint of heart. With this knowledge comes the innate urge to take responsibility, an unpleasant prospect for many. No matter your level of interest in the workings of the world around you and you're your commitment to making it a better place, once you take the red pill, you can never go back and see the world in the same way . . . .

Welcome, red pills

Every day I watch dozens of school children in my neighborhood suffer the ill effects of an oppressive medical system that preys upon them. Sound like too strong a comment to begin a book? Perhaps it is. But in my 20 plus years of service to the community as a dedicated Chiropractic Physician, I feel the time has come for drastic measures by parents who've had enough. Compiled studies show that *autism* has increased as much as 3,000 times from where it was 75 years ago, and *childhood cancer* is the leading killer of children ages 3 to 14. Over the past 7 years autism rose a staggering 273% in California following their whooping cough vaccination program. Autism, a subclinical form of *encephalitis (brain damage due to brain swelling), was hardly noticeable in America until the advent of mandatory vaccination programs.* Consider the following statistical information on autism:

One in 10,000 births were autistic in the 1970's
One in 500 in the 1980's
One in 100 in the 1990's
One in 86 in 2003 (United Kingdom Study)

The only thing that could create such a drastic change in our population, to make a form of mental retardation almost commonplace in less than 50 years time, is the systematic neurological poisoning of the population. By a simple process of elimination, the common denominator acting as the toxic agent in the varying communities around the globe in which we find autism, is most obviously the array of toxic poisons found in every medical vaccine. Our global autism pandemic was most certainly caused by the high levels of mercury and other lethal toxins injected directly into the bloodstream of practically 95% of our population through forced vaccines.

Some people are asking why, attempting to find the "hidden" meaning to this tragedy. But most researchers are asking the *wrong questions.* The fact is simple. The bulk of medically orientated care of our children does not work, especially when we consider the practice of medical "prevention" through vaccines. It never has worked, and to the contrary, medical "care" is the primary reason our society is as sick as it is today. To date the World Health Organization reports over 30 countries where the general health and well-being of its people far exceed that of North Americans. Considering that North America is one of the wealthier continents on the globe, doesn't this raise a brow of suspicion? This text will attempt to explain why to you in a step by step fashion, backed by solid research to further expose the fraud that has been pushed upon us all, especially over the past three decades.

Here is what you can expect to discover from this text, so keep on reading if you are interested:

1. There is absolutely **NO PROOF ANYWHERE** that vaccinated children are healthier than non-vaccinated children. In fact, the exact opposite is true.

2. Despite what your pediatrician may tell you, there is absolutely **NO PROOF ANYWHERE** that the party line statement, "vaccine benefits outweigh the risks" is true. In fact, there is a ton of evidence pointing in the opposite direction.

3. There is **NO PROOF ANYWHERE** that vaccinations are safe.

4. Vaccinations cause illness, death and disease.

5. There are no long-term safety studies completed on vaccines.

6. Vaccines cause crib death, autism, brain damage and childhood cancer.

7. Deaths from old childhood diseases were due to poor sanitation and improper public hygiene, and were mostly gone long before the onset of vaccination programs.

8. Vaccines contain lethal toxins and poisons.

9. Childhood diseases actually strengthen the immune system naturally.

10. Vaccines are responsible for the astronomical rise in spinal meningitis and encephalitis over the past five decades.

11. Vaccines are strongly linked to learning difficulties, hyperactivity and many forms of mental retardation.

12. You can legally avoid vaccinations in any state regardless of the "law."

This text is a simple compilation and review of the facts which have been available for a long time. Aside from my private natural healing practice of Chiropractic, I have not done any personal research projects to support the data which already exists. There really is no need to do so anyway, since the data which exists is still undeniable. I have however, read hundreds of major texts available on the subject over the years, as well as hundreds of the references which formed those texts. This made me come to the conclusion that a summary text such as this one is not only beneficial, but vitally necessary for people to access. The books explaining the research compiled for the anti-vaccine issue are many in number, yet few explain things in a precise, direct classroom style manner, as does this book. Many are laden with statistical facts and charts that the layman may have difficulty sifting through, and thus fully understand. My hope is that this book will serve as a guideline for further inquiry and personal study into the workings of what I call the *Medical cartel*, a now complicated network of medical professionals, government officials and pharmaceutical companies, who exist solely for profit off an unassuming, unsuspecting naive and brainwashed public. This book also provides legal strategies for relief of oppressive vaccination laws.

Oh sure, you can read all the mainstream pamphlets put out by the Medical cartel, and they are sure to tell you the exact opposite of what you will learn in this text. Who are you going to believe? I submit that you get all the facts, and decide what the truth is for yourself using *common sense*; a commodity of American civilization which has become terribly wounded. People need to wake up to the realization that private interest groups, such as pharmaceutical companies, the American Medical Association, and the politicians writhing their hands to obtain pay backs, submit mile high piles of *JUNK SCIENCE* to both the people and government, creating political agendas through paranoia which generate huge profits. People also need to wake up to the realization that whenever private research groups complete investigations on the wares of the Medical cartel, primarily drugs and vaccines, the results are not as colorful. Often they are quite disastrous.

Before we get started with this material, understand that it will most definitely upset you. Not in any way do I intend to criticize any particular medical professional by the writings herein. I stand firm on my belief that most medical doctors are good and hard working people, who have nothing but the best intentions in mind for their patients. But then again, most medical professionals, especially doctors, are vastly misguided. I have met many people who, once presented with a book the likes such as this one, fall into a eulogy of medical fire and brimstone; *"How dare you say this! I had a loving Auntie who died of tuberculosis! I had a brother who was totally paralyzed from polio! The Salk vaccine saved us all from the same fate, probably even you! I had a cousin who was in an iron lung from pertussis! How could you be so ungrateful for what our modern medicine has provided for us!!!!??"* On and on and on they go, preaching the doctrine of the medical religion, and promising damnation for those who don't comply. They base their strong emotionally charged support for vaccinations on fraudulent statistical information promoted by the medical cartel and government officials. Some don't know any better and are just caught in the *matrix*. Some do and purposely keep the fraud moving forward.

Fact is, the medical profession is vitally necessary in our world. My son had an accident where he required many stitches, and I was eternally grateful for the skilled hands of the caring plastic surgeon, who came off his fishing boat to call on my emergency. My son has no scars due to this man. When I was nine, my appendix nearly burst. If not for the caring doctors and hospital staff, who performed an emergency appendectomy at 3:15 AM, I would not be writing this book today. I have known cases of children with brain dysfunction, where medication was absolutely necessary to bring them out of their inner cage, and function happily and productively in the world. Certainly, **with due consideration**, medicine has its' place. But this book is not about that. It is also not about grieving for the tragedies of people who have experienced hardships at the face of some disease process. This book is about an oppressive system of medical government now out of control in America, and it is certainly about rethinking the germ theory into a more plausible, logical theory of true health care, not merely *disease care*. The unfortunate truth is that, despite all its' credits, modern medicine has done far more damage to our society than it has good, and should always be procured with extreme caution.

If you believe medical care has helped your child, this book will make you think twice about your particular story. Once again, medicine does have its' place in this world. When allowed to expand outside the realm of crisis care however, in which medicine has more than exceeded its' boundaries, the net result on our nation has been more than disastrous. It is an out right crime unlike any other of recorded history.

Let me ask you a very serious question, parent to parent. What would you do to an individual, or a group of individuals who purposely caused physical harm to your precious child, all for their own profit and gain? Would you call the police? Hire a lawyer and begin a serious lawsuit? Take matters into your own hands and go after them with a club? Now suppose you do any of these things and get chastised by the "authorities," arrested, and have your child taken away from you, only to have the same harmful process repeated on them forcefully by these same individuals. What would you do?

The better question to ask today I suppose is, "*what are you going to do?*" This scenario is real, and it is happening in America right now as you read this text. The DCF (department of children and families) in States around the country are taking children from their parents, claiming that the parents are negligent for not providing these children with a brand of medical care they, "*the State*", deem is best for the child. An even better question to ask is, how can this all be happening? We still have God given, creator endowed unalienable rights in this country, and many people don't realize this as the DCF walks off with their children and forcefully medicates them against their will. This is primarily because parents are asking the **WRONG QUESTIONS!** Everyone just assumes that germs cause disease, vaccines and other medicines are of the purest quality and actually work, and that the local and State governments have the right to do what they do. This book will show you that 95% of the time any government agency acts, they **DO NOT HAVE THE AUTHORITY** to do what they do, especially when it comes to forcefully medicating anyone, let alone a person's child. I will also show you how to ask the **RIGHT QUESTIONS**, and move forward against any corrupt bureaucrat with the proper skills and paperwork, like a bull dog rather than a frightened sheep.

This book was written because the author has finally reached his speed limit for what he is able to watch. I can no longer stand idly by as more and more defenseless children become victims of mindless and villainous vaccination policies. The compiled research which so obviously points to vaccinations being responsible for autism, childhood cancer, crib death (sudden infant death syndrome, or SIDS), allergies, asthma, ADHD, mental retardation and other forms of childhood brain damage is staggering! Yet the money powers that be in the AMA and the medical / pharmaceutical cartel relentlessly lie, cheat, and fraudulently present research which obfuscates the point, that they are responsible for mostly every disorder they are attempting to alleviate. They control how the media reports them, the MD's who act as good foot soldiers underneath them, and the politicians who support their fraud. The AMA and its' associated pharmaceutical companies (the center of operations for the medical cartel) have been the number one political contribution group for decades. This should also raise a brow, since they spend billions on lobbying annually to make mega trillions in return. They have become so powerful that they feel no one, not government, moral society, or even God has authority over them. When anyone questions their motives, they simply don't answer in an air of condescension, and laugh all the way to the bank.

Many people are familiar with how the radar detector manufacturers, who sell a myriad of detection devices to the general public, also manufacture and sell the actual radar devices to the police. This beautiful scenario helps them create profits out of thin air. Upgrades in police radar devices are followed shortly by upgrades in the public's choices of radar detection devices. It goes on and on and on. But this is exactly how the AMA and its' army of medical profiteers thrive. The medical cartel owns the CDC (a federal organization called the *center for disease control*), and many other federal agencies. They have no problem what so ever in creating diseases and disease panic, spread through the media and legislated by various puppet agencies. I will show you how they have systematically created many a disease panic, using their powers in the media and the FDA to provide mass panic, followed by their own brand of "cure" and vaccine. I will also show you how they have falsified research, tricking the public and lawmakers into believing their vaccines and medicines have actually helped society. The brain washed aspect of our society then runs for these cures. State health departments are offered more cash in "federal aid" if they comply with appropriate law making campaigns to support the medical cartels' lies. This happens every day of our lives.

When I was a boy, our doctor was my home town's only MD for years. He was a dedicated and humble man, who believed that there was nothing good diet and rest could not cure. During this time, he told me that "vaccines were poison and good for nothing." He refused to administer them to anyone. Despite this, I went through the standard propaganda training through school that disease is something you catch from the outside world, usually in the form of some foreign body called a "germ." I entered college with high aspirations of becoming a medical doctor and learning how to heal people. But something happened during my Junior year that made me take a more serious look at medicine.

I had slit my big toe on a friends slate step, running up to his pool. It was quite a bloody mess. After the bandaging, my knowledge made me insist on a trip to a physician who would give me a tetanus shot, and all agreed this was a wise decision of a smart young man on his way to becoming a good doctor. So I went to go see the doctor, he administered the tetanus vaccine, and I fell into anaphylactic shock on his treatment room floor a few seconds later.

Although I did not have the standard "out of body experience" you hear of in most "almost died" stories, I was indeed, almost dead. I remember having a clear sense in my blacked out state that I could leave this world here and now. Although I blacked out, what I saw in front of me was nothing like black. It was more like spiraling and sparkling lights swirling around me. I felt an almost immediate sense of panic that I might be permanently detached from my physical body, and realized that I could not locate my physical substance anywhere in my perception. I may very well have been called into the void, but a loud voice emanating from within me said firmly, *"NO!"* I realized then that it was not my time to leave, and I felt myself gently sink back into a more cohesive awareness of my physical form. Then I awoke, collapsed on the floor (I was sitting on an examining table for the shot) with two doctors, a nurse and a receptionist nervously and intently starring at me. One doctor immediately re-took my blood pressure. The cuff was already on my arm.

"What happened," I asked them.

"We've been trying to revive you for 5 minutes," the doctor replied. "Your blood pressure practically went down to zero." This was 1977, before the days of high mal-practice which causes doctors to persistently lie to their patients. In today's world with the exact same circumstances, no doctor in their right mind would tell you the truth, especially just after administering you a vaccine. I was grateful for his information, and left thinking I had simply passed out due to anxiety centered around receiving a shot. The funny thing was however, that I wasn't the slightest bit anxious about it. That was the last time I would have an injection of any kind other than lidocaine at the dentist.

This experience slowly but surely changed my life. I decided to leave pre-med and go into secondary education. I taught High School Biology and Chemistry for two years deciding whether or not I wanted to pursue a career in medicine. I actually did become accepted into a medical school in NYC, simultaneously with my acceptance to the local Chiropractic college. Through my 4 plus years at NY Chiropractic college, then located on Long Island, I was aware that half of my 110 classmates were there because they figured there was no chance they would be accepted into medical school. Although I mostly kept it to myself that I choose a career in Chiropractic over medicine, close friends I did tell of my story could scarcely believe I would do such a thing. MD's were considered then the crème de la crème of doctors. They had all the privileges and insurance rights. They drove the big cars and made the big bucks without any problems after graduation. As a DC (doctor of Chiropractic), at best one was considered a second class kind of doctor who has to educate his patients about what he does. What a foolish burden I had laid upon myself!

Well, nearly 25 years after first walking through those doors at NY Chiropractic college, I still have no regrets. In fact, every year I am able to serve people with natural, wholesome Chiropractic care, which is true **HEALTH CARE** rather than the disease care perpetrated by the medical profession, I feel eternally blessed. This book will describe to you many natural remedies and modalities as alternatives to the popular medical pills, potions and lotions.

I have been watching this medical profession very closely since the time of my childhood. We are dealing with a demon here of colossal proportions. You should never take this single fact for granted. If they are not stopped *here, and now*, they will grow to encompass and control our lives and the lives of our children in ways you may now think unimaginable. Believe me, they have only just begun. Each of you reading this text must stand up and fight for your right to choose what is best for your child and yourself. If you don't know your rights, you don't have any. If you continually sit idly by without asking questions, you will loose all your rights, even the ones you may think you have.

Like the government, this medical cartel uses specific planned out modes of psychological mind control to frighten people into "voluntary" compliance. The propaganda you have absorbed in your life up to now will no doubt come to the forefront as you read these pages, coaxing you to be skeptical and loyal to what you have been told. Most people will read these pages and automatically sense, from a higher portion of themselves beyond their conditioning, that there is truth here. During the congressional hearings on the relationship between autism and vaccines, lead by congressman Butron in April of 1999, everyone could see on CSPAN how the MD puppets the medical cartel placed there were having a lot of trouble denying the facts that autism has been created by vaccines. But they still present fraudulent research promoted and paid for by the medical cartel itself, assuring everyone that vaccines are safe. Yeah right! DPT and MMR are safe, even though Europe and Japan banned them in 1975, and endless pages of research compiled by organizations other than the medical cartel say otherwise. Despite this, the AMA insists on our compliance and trust, stating that they will "look into the matter." In the meantime, take two more shots and call me in the morning with brain damage.

The unfortunate end result of all this bickering is that people who don't understand the argument, which accounts for 90% of the worlds population, wind up defaulting on to the advice of their brain washed MD or pediatrician, who assures them that no matter what they are hearing out there, vaccines and other medical treatments are safe, and anyone who opposes such a view is some kind of terrorist lunatic. It amazes me that this can be so, when all a parent has to do is read the packet insert of vaccines, which explains the risks and side effects. The only logical question to ask your pediatrician after reading that packet insert is, "how can you say these are safe?" The MD may answer, "well, it's certainly safer than the risk of becoming infected with the disease," but I assure you, this text will prove how that is absolute nonsense. There is nothing but truth and facts on these pages; ones you can use to free yourself, your family and community.

The time has come for serious action if you want to protect yourself and your family. You must learn all the facts about what is really going on out there. You must now become a voice; and as loud a voice as you possibly can. A revolution against the medical profession and cartel, who have become their own form of government, more powerful than you may imagine, is well overdue. I ask you to join this cause here and now, with the heart of a lion and the faith of a child. Winston Churchill once said that it is far better to choose to fight when there is a slim chance of winning, then to have to fight when there is no chance at all. We are at that time of critical choice. Choose wisely. Your family's future very much depends on it.

Dr. William Palaski-Trebing and
son Alexander William
29 September, 2000

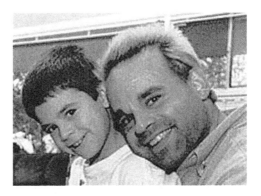

"I believe that more than 90% of modern medicine could disappear from the face of the Earth—doctor, hospital, drug and equipment—and the effect on our health would be immediate and beneficial."

Robert Mendelsohn, MD (in loving memory)
author of Confessions of a Medical Heretic

Rest in peace old friend. Your voice of truth continues through all those you inspired. The torch is still brightly lit, and I believe one day we will all be free.

Chapter One
Medical Mayhem

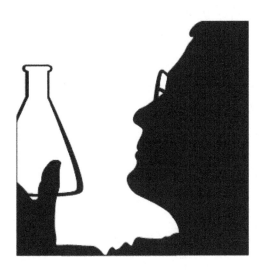

Are germs a causative factor in disease? For most of you the very question must seem absurd. You have probably never been confronted with this kind of question or even thought about considering it, because somehow through a series of some very interesting historical frauds, this idea that germs cause disease has come to the forefront of people's thinking around the world, despite a massive amount of valid research to oppose it. This research all points to disease being something we have done to ourselves, rather than something we are invaded by. What the medical cartel calls disease is nothing more than a natural process of toxic elimination. The more toxic you become over the years, the more profound your eliminative process. Standardized medicine categorizes the symptoms of this eliminative process in neat little packages, and this is what they call their myriad of diseases. They then provide chemicals which alter the body in ways to shut off this process of detoxification and elimination. But in all actuality, from the wisest point of view on health you can find, *the only cure for what is happening to you when you are toxic is your disease.* Just think for a moment of what disease means. Dis-Ease. The body is out of balance and out of its normal harmony, and it is attempting to work its' way back to homeostasis.

What exactly is *immunity?* People have been taught that it is the body's way to fight germs, but nothing can be further from the truth. In a medical sense, all immunity means is that you possess a particular set of antibodies which are supposed to correspond to a particular disease. That's all it means! Being immune from the disease does not mean you will never get the disease. Your immune system is designed to eliminate the accumulation of dead, morbid matter which is highly toxic. What exactly does this mean, accumulated morbid matter? In a large sense, it has to do with the life we live, the air we breathe, the water we drink, and especially it is concerned with the foods we eat and the stress we experience. Our bodies are quite versatile and can accumulate a ton of these stressors before anything really happens. But there comes a point where the body says *"I'm mad as hell, and I'm not going to take it any more!"* This is when it begins its' eliminative process and you feel yourself becoming *"sick."* A body that can do this, mustering up enough vitality to throw off toxicity, is indeed healthy. This process of throwing off waste and toxicity is what modern medicine calls disease.

Medicine places groups of symptoms together to form their dreaded diseases, but these symptoms are exactly what your body needs to become healthy and pure again. Symptoms are the open doors to restoring health and vitality. Medicine however chooses to close those doors by eliminating the symptoms. When this is done over an extended period of time, we enter the realm of chronic and disastrous disease.

If you are taking medications to shut off these avenues of wellness the medical people call symptoms, you are shutting off the only avenues of vitality you have to burn off and eliminate toxicity and poison. On top of this, you are introducing far worse poisons into your body, which the body now has to work harder to overcome and eliminate. If this is done repeatedly over a number of years, death soon follows.

The medical professions' claim to fame on disease prevention has always been the revered vaccine. But what exactly is a vaccine? I'll bet your medical doctor has never told you they contain rotten proteinaceous wastes in the form of dead animal tissue, along with a myriad of cancer producing stabilizers and neutralizing agents. What's worse is they inject this junk directly into the blood stream of would be healthy children. It's not like the body has several lines of defense through the digestive system before these toxins reach the blood. They shock the body with a direct hit. This concept, above all others, is absolutely insane and continues to defy logic, year after deadly year. The DEW (department of health, education and welfare) used to print in their parents guide that the decision to vaccinate your child is yours alone to make. It should concern everyone reading this book that this statement is no longer in print.

Ask yourself, what induced you to vaccinate your child? What makes you continue with vaccines? Most parents say it is fear of their children becoming ill and dying from catching a disease. Others add it is the responsible thing to do. I will prove to you in this book that you are doing a much greater harm to yourself and your child by vaccinating medically, as opposed to not doing so. The issues which surround these ideas of requiring the medical profession to take care of us are more a matter of propaganda and brain washing than established fact.

There is also a general misconception that all MD's agree with the idea of vaccination. Here are some quotes which prove otherwise.

The Surgeon General, Leonard Sheele MD spoke before the AMA in 1955, stating:

"No batch of vaccine can be proven safe before it is given to children."

In 1967, James Shannon MD of the NIH (national institute of health) said:

"The only safe vaccine is a vaccine that is never used."

Hugh Fudenberg, MD, one of the most respected immunogeneticists in the world, compiled research on Alzheimer's disease concerning the years 1970 to 1980. He stated this at a public meeting in 1997:

"The chances of getting Alzheimer's disease is ten times higher if an individual has had five consecutive flu shots between 1970 and 1980, than if they had just one, two or no shots."

In 1926, the Journal of the American Medical Association (JAMA) noted:

"In regions in which there is no organized vaccination of the population, general paralysis [to polio] is rare. It is impossible to deny a connection between vaccination and the encephalitis [brain damage] which follows it."

H. Mullen writes in the book, "Murder by Injection:"

"... vaccine is the cause of more diseases and sufferings than anything I can name. Such diseases as cancer, syphilis, cold sores, and many other disease conditions are the direct result of vaccination. Yet, in the state of Virginia and many other states parents are compelled to submit their children to this procedure while the medical profession not only receives it pay for this service, but also makes splendid and prospective clients for the future ..."

Vaccines are not only recognized for some of their known side effects, such as anaphylactic shock, seizures, brain damage, learning disabilities and autism. They are responsible for many chronic and degenerative diseases, such as arthritis, colitis and cancer.

J. Anthony Morris, Ph.D. of the FDA virology vaccine lab & department of biostatistics and biologics said in 1987:

"I am against mandating compulsory vaccination laws, because I have met no one in government who has the wisdom to mandate to another person what that person should do with his child. I have been in government some 30 years and I can tell you, that when I sat in the halls of those persons concerned with setting policies for vaccination procedures in this country, that I was never impressed there was a great depository of wisdom in that room. There just wasn't. I believe that the person who is far more capable for determining what happens to a child is the parent of that child, rather than some bureaucrat who sits around a table in Washington ..."

But as we speak, there is a big push happening in federal government for compulsory mandated vaccines, pushed for by the AMA and pharmaceutical lobbying efforts.

Dr. Morris continues:

" . . . when I left the FDA in 1976, there was no technique available to measure reliably and consistently neurotoxicity or potency of the vaccines then in use. Today, 11 years later the situation remains essentially the same."

The connection between compulsory vaccines and autism can no longer be denied. The enhanced public awareness of this fact is brought to light by parents all over the globe today. New evidence shows that 1 in 100 children are suffering from some form of autism, neurological problem, behavioral and / or immune system dysfunction. Talk about epidemics! After 15 years the media finally has taken notice, placing a U.S. congressional hearing on television in April of 1999. There we saw the efforts of a few honest congressmen and courageous medical doctors whose independent, multi-disciplinary approach to investigating the biological mechanism of vaccine induced autism, is serving as a counter weight to the steadfast denials by infectious disease "specialists", and government health officials defending the current compulsory vaccination policies. It made me ill to see how these supporters of the present vaccine system twist reality. Colleen Boyle, a representative for the CDC, read a prepared statement denying any connection between autism and vaccines. Congressman Burton asked her if she thought it was a conflict of interest for the same people who were funded by the vaccine manufacturers, to be on the Advisory Board of the CDC, making decisions about which vaccines should be given to American children. Boyle did not answer. Burton repeated the question, but Boyle was speechless. Boyle's sudden paralysis of the vocal chords during this moment speaks volumes to our cause; *that vaccines are promoted for profit and a means of controlling the public, not for public gain.*

What I have actually discovered from my personal associations with many good MD's, is that there is a generalized ambivalence regarding the subject of vaccination. They know in their hearts that the process is totally wrong and harmful, but many keep quiet for fear of becoming the outcast, or worse, the de-licensed. Let's now look into the facts about vaccines that make them feel this way.

"Every doctor will allow a colleague to decimate a whole countryside sooner than violate the bond of professional etiquette by giving him away."

George Bernard Shaw

Chapter Two
The Poisoned Needle

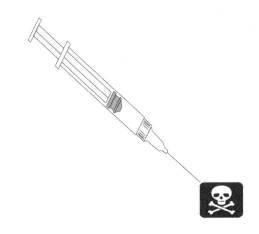

"There has never been a single vaccine in this country [the USA] that has ever been submitted to a controlled scientific study. They never took a group of 100 people who were candidates for a vaccine, gave 50 of them a vaccine and left the other 50 alone to measure the outcome. And since that hasn't been done, that means if you want to be kind, you will call vaccines an unproven remedy. If you want to be accurate, you'll call people who give vaccines 'quacks.'"

Robert Mendelsohn, MD

Party line #1:	Vaccines create immunity in the people who receive them, by placing foreign viruses or bacteria through injection into their blood streams. This gives the person a weakened form of the disease, which stimulates antibody production to protect the person if and when the real disease ever comes along.

"The medical authorities keep lying. Vaccination is a disaster to the immune system. It actually causes a lot of illnesses and brain damage. We are changing our genetic code through vaccination."
Guylaine Lanctot, MD author of Medical Mafia

Mostly everyone has been taught the basic premises of vaccination. The above party line sounds very nice, but it has *no basis in medical or scientific fact.* In fact, the entire connection between antibody production and immunity (in the sense that you will not get the disease you are being vaccinated for) to any allegedly contagious disease does not exist. The packet inserts

55

provided with each vaccine do not even state a child will receive protection from any particular disease. All they state is that the shot will increase antibody counts, and this statement is virtually meaningless. We will go more in depth on antibody production after our discussion of vaccines.

"My data proves that the studies used to support vaccinations are so flawed that it is impossible to say if vaccination provides a net benefit to anyone or to society in general. This question can only be determined by proper studies which have never been performed."
John Classen, MD medical researcher

"I found that the whole vaccine business was indeed a gigantic hoax. Most doctors are convinced that they are useful, but if you look at the proper statistics you will realize that this is not so."
Archie Kalokerinos, MD medical researcher

"There is a great deal of evidence to prove that vaccinations of children does far more harm than good."
J. Anthony Morris, Ph. D.
Chief vaccine control officer for the FDA—

p.s.—he was fired the day after he made this public statement in the early 1970's. He later fought and got his job back just in time to be a major critic of then president Gerald Ford's swine flu vaccination campaign, which killed thousands of people. For doing this he again, lost his job.

The basic premises on which the vaccination theory above is built on, can be separated into four categories, or better said, assumptions:

1. Vaccines are safe.
2. Vaccines are effective in what they are supposed to do.
3. Vaccines are responsible for the decline of infectious diseases we have witnessed over the past 100 years.
4. Vaccines are the only way to prevent epidemic outbreaks.

Every single one of these assumptions created by the medical cartel is absolutely false. Lets begin with #1, *vaccines are safe.*

Vaccines are so safe, that the federal government had to set up a separate service to handle all the reporting and complaints of vaccine related damages. The service is called **VAERS**, which stands for Vaccine Adverse Event Reporting System. VAERS received a total of 54,072 reports of adverse reactions to vaccines, which includes disease, injury and at least 471 deaths, following vaccination in a 43 month period from April of 1990 to November 0f 1993. At least 1,094 deaths were reported from 1990 to 1997. According to these reports alone, vaccines have killed over 3 children per week.

Vaccines are so safe, that the popular magazine *Mothering*, reported in 1998:

"Approximately one-half of the hundreds of parents who call our office each month report that their child became autistic shortly after receiving a vaccination."

Vaccines are so safe, that not one private insurance company in the world will insure them. You can get life insurance, car insurance, medical insurance, disability insurance . . . . the list is endless. But you can't get vaccine insurance anywhere on the planet. Insurance companies say they will insure most anything, with the exception of damage of life and property due to *acts of God, Nuclear War, and Vaccinations.* Isn't this a curious fact? Vaccines are so safe, that in the early 1990's the federal government had to administer a torte limitation on damage pay outs concerning vaccine related lawsuits. A torte limitation is a damage limitation on the amount of money that can be paid out for said damages in court. The only time that torte limitations are installed is when the number of claims, and the amount of money being paid out is overburdening the industry which is a victim of the suits. In this case, it would seem that we are obviously talking about the pharmaceutical industry. But the federal government has totally absolved the pharmaceutical companies from any and all damages due to vaccines. It is usually the federal or State government who pays out vaccination related lawsuit damages, and we will discuss this in more detail later.

Senate bills S733 and S732 talk about the national vaccine injury compensation act and program. Aside from other things, they attempted and failed with these bills to set up a national vaccine registry, with all of your personal history and personal information on it. Good thing this was shot down, but be certain that it will raise its' ugly head again and again until the people scream they have had enough. The now senator (dear Lord!) Hillary health care plan is nothing more than a collection of oppressive laws, masked under the disguise of added privileges, that would allow pharmaceutical companies and the medical cartel to further control your life. Her bill led to these senate bills, and was the initial information gathering, health registry type of bill in America. Everyone should be very concerned that Hillary is now a State senator. The goal is simply to force compliance with the medical cartel. If you do not get vaccinated, they would automatically know of it and deny you plane travel, hotel stays, tax rebates . . . . you name it. Stay aware of this one and be sure it never gets passed.

If vaccines are so safe, why then in America are claims being filed, quite literally every day, by parents whose children have become brain damaged, and harmed in many other ways following a vaccine? According to the *Health Research Council*, an organization which monitors federal vaccine damage programs, between 1986 and 1992 alone there were 4,569 claims filed against the pharmaceutical companies that create the vaccines and doctors which administer them. So far, 928 have been paid to the tune of 369 million in damages. This comes out, approximately, to over 600 claims per year, or two per day. And they say vaccines are safe? What's wrong with this picture? You should further understand that this is not a private insurer paying out these damage claims. Remember, no company in the world will insure vaccines, not even to the medical cartel. So guess who's paying them out? You are, with your tax dollars. State and federal government have exonerated the pharmaceutical companies from blame, and use tax money to pay out damage claims.

The medical cartel has net over 5 billion dollars in profits from vaccines since 1981, and this is what they admit to. The figure is most likely quite a bit higher than this in reality. Keep in mind, this is an admitted *net profit of over 5 billion.* The gross income is obviously an even greater number. So then, with 5 billion dollars in profits, the federal government also decides to indemnify them against any damages by covering their claims costs with your tax dollars. Further, they provide them with sizable grants to commence free vaccine programs around the country, as well as in foreign lands. Just recently they have also installed a torte limitation on the amount of money that they will pay out to YOU if your child has vaccine damage. WOW! This is a pretty good deal! Have you ever heard of any one company or organization being offered so many amazing and protective privileges? It is like the federal government has insured them to make money no matter what happens. Very curious, indeed. You should be asking why this is so.

Now lets move on to #2. *Vaccines are effective in what they are supposed to do.*

Let us begin this discussion with the anatomy of a vaccine. You will be told by the pharmaceutical companies that they are live or attenuated (weakened) viruses or bacteria, sometimes in the form of foreign blood along with certain carrying agents, stabilizers and other additives that supposedly help stimulate further antibody production. Lets add here that none of these substances are indigenous to the body. The form that these viruses, bacteria and other additives assume in a vaccine are complex (large) proteins. Proteins of this size are never found in the bloodstream, because they are digested into smaller, less toxic components before they enter. But you are not eating these proteins. You are having them injected directly into your blood stream, and this is very bad for the body. These heavy and large proteins making their way to the nervous system and brain are argument enough for a causative factor in brain damage and nervous system disorders, but it gets far worse. We are only warming up here.

Proteins in the blood, especially large polypeptides like the ones you receive from vaccines, are a most unnatural and dangerous circumstance. They are simply too big to be in the blood, and this makes for a ridiculously toxic chemical circumstance. The body uses protein building blocks, called amino acids, to build proteins naturally. Protein food is broken down in the stomach and absorbed into the blood as these simple amino acids. Large proteins in the blood putrefy, which means they actually rot there, in the same way that meat goes rancid over time when not refrigerated. This produces a myriad of toxic by-products in the blood, most of which are carcinogenic. The body has to work very hard to detoxify these proteins. When they build up in the blood they can easily overload the system into a healing crisis of some shape and form. Run off to your local MD, and you'll get a nice diagnosis of the same shape and form. He'll try to shut off your symptoms with a potion, pill or lotion, which adds fuel to the fire your body is attempting to put out.

Haven't you ever wondered why an otherwise beautiful and healthy child drops dead, or develops almost immediate brain damage after receiving a vaccine? There have been an array of TV shows over the past 10 years that cover "bad lots" of the DPT vaccine, and raise many questions on vaccine safety that are well overdue. But they are only scratching the surface of what needs to be discussed. The reason vaccines are the scourge they have become, is primarily due to their unbelievably high level of toxicity. For example, the *DPT shot*, which is receiving a ton of press these days (25 years overdue according to Europe and Japan however. I wonder if it makes any difference that this shot is manufactured in the USA?), contains amongst other things these wonderful additives, according to its' packet insert:

    a.   *Formaldehyde* (embalming fluid for dead folks)—a class "A" carcinogen according to the FDA.

    b.   *Mercury*—one of the most potent neurotoxins known to man, linked by endless research with dementia and nervous system breakdown disorders like multiple sclerosis, Alzheimer's and Parkinson's diseases.

    c.   *Aluminum phosphate*—added by the pharmaceutical company to further enhance antibody production. Also a potent carcinogen and linked by research to nervous system breakdown disorders like Parkinson's disease and Alzheimer's disease.

The *polio shot* is not any better:

a. *Aluminum potassium sulfate*—creates same aluminum nervous system damage as above.
b. *Thimerosal*—a mercury derivative that is as toxic as mercury.(a component in over 50 vaccines!)
c. *Monkey kidney cell culture*—a monkey's kidney is injected with what is assumed to be polio virus and other toxic stabilizers. This is continued until the monkey sickens and nearly dies. The cell culture from that sick kidney is now taken out and mixed with carrying agents.
d. *Albumin*—large polypeptide (protein) from egg whites.
e. *Antibiotics*
f. *Calf serum*—I have called, and have yet to find anyone at the CDC who can tell me why calf serum is in this vaccine.

The *MMR (measles, mumps and rubella) shot* contains thimerosal, plus;

a. *Cultured cells of an infected Chick embryo*
b. *Neomycin*—one of the most recognized potent immunosuppressant antibiotics made.

The *diphtheria shot* contains:

a. *Blood from an infected horse*—the horse receives repeated injection of supposed diphtheria sputum with toxic carrying agents. When the horse is so sick it can't stand anymore, its' blood is drawn and used in this vaccine.
b. The same carrying agents as DPT shot plus highly toxic thimerosal.

The *small pox shot* contains thimerosal and toxic carrying agents, plus:

a. *Infected Calf serum*—a calf is cut with sharp blades on the belly. Alleged small pox virus and dirt is then placed in the wound. The pus is then taken, mixed with glycerin and used in the vaccine.

Once again, keep in mind that we are not talking about taking these products orally. They are injected into the blood, shocking the hell out of the body and usually sending it into a state of crisis. This is done to boost your immunity? Has anyone ever had their doctor tell them the risks of placing these incredibly toxic substances directly into the blood flow? Why not ask your pediatrician next time you see her?

Here are some more fine ingredients (a.k.a. lethal poisons) ubiquitous to most of the 74 vaccines your child is expected to receive before the age of 6:

Ammonium sulfate(salt): Gastrointestinal, liver and nerve poison.

Beta-propiolactone: Causes liver and stomach cancer; lung irritant.

Genetically modified yeast

Animal, bacterial and viral DNA: Can create genetic mutations.

Latex rubber: Anaphylactic shock and death.

MSG: Reproductive malformations and allergies.

Aluminum: Alzheimer's disease, dementia, seizures and coma.

Formaldehyde: Linked to leukemia, brain and colon cancer.

Polysorbate 60: Proven carcinogen.

Tri(n) butylphosphate: Kidney and nerve poison.

Glutaraldehyde: Poison, causes birth defects.

Gelatin: Allergies.

Gentamicin sulfate and polymyxin B: Allergies.

Mercury: Historically one of the most potent toxins known to exist. Very minute amounts create nerve and brain damage. By age 6 vaccinated children receive 125 times the safe limit of mercury set by the Environmental Protection Agency. Mercury moves easily across the placenta to growing fetuses.

Neomycin sulfate: Interferes with vitamin B6 absorption, causing epilepsy and mental retardation.

Phenol(carbolic acid)/phenoxyethanol or ethylene glycol: Antifreeze for cars. Toxic to all living cells.

Human and animal cells: Source is aborted human fetal tissue, pig blood, horse blood, rabbit brain, dog kidney, cow heart, sheep blood.

Borax: Used as ant killer.

Considering the immensely toxic nature of the mercury derivative thimerosal, here is a quote from medical historian Harris L. Coulter, Ph.D.

"A major cause of the Roman Empire's decline, after 6 centuries of world dominance was its replacement of stone aqueducts by lead pipes for the transport and supply of drinking water. Roman engineers, the best in the world, turned their fellow citizens into neurological cripples. Today our own "best and brightest" with the best intentions, achieve the same end through childhood vaccination programs yielding the modern scurges of hyperactivity, learning disabilities, autism, appetite disorders, and impulsive violence."

Another obvious problem with the administration of vaccines, is that you are overriding your bodies natural defenses to toxic input. With every shot, you weaken your own body's ability to care for itself, especially if you receive these shots in succession. Reading from the *PDR* (physicians desk reference) and the *organic consumer* reports regarding vaccines:

".... injections of foreign substances like viruses, toxins and foreign proteins into the blood stream by a vaccination have been associated with diseases and disorders of the blood, brain, nervous system and skin. Rare diseases such as atypical measles and monkey fever, as well as such well known disorders, such as premature aging, and allergies have been associated with vaccines. Also linked to immunizations are such well known diseases as cancer, leukemia, paralysis, multiple sclerosis, arthritis, and sudden infant death syndrome ..."

Haven't they just said it all right there? Why would anyone succumb to this level of risk?

Large protein molecules in the blood cannot be digested, since the blood contains no proteolytic (protein eating) enzymes to do such a thing. As stated earlier, this protein quite literally rots in your blood, decomposing much like a dead animal left on your doorstep by your cat. This decomposition of proteins now releases an array of toxic products which are floating freely throughout your body. You have become one large toxic soup.

These toxic products released into the blood from rotting proteins are some of the most toxic, and vile substances known to mankind. If you are familiar with biochemistry, you'll recognize them as **indols, phenols, creatinines, ptomaines, and glucamines.** One of the ptomaines released persistently into the blood from vaccines is *cadaverine*, found exclusively in dead bodies (hence the name), and one of the key components found in *rigor mortis*. Something tells me you never read about this in the NY Times, or heard this on the watered down DPT stories on TV.

It is even a bigger crime that the medical profession knows of these toxic side effects of vaccines. Thank God for indemnity, otherwise they would never admit to any of them. To cover their butts in court, they always say that the risks were clearly printed out on the packet inserts. You should have read them. For DPT, the packet insert admits the following side effects:

a. Severe temperature, 105 degrees or greater
b. Collapse
c. Prolonged prostration and shock like state
d. Screaming episodes (indicates brain damage)
e. Autism
f. Hyperactivity
g. Isolated convulsions
h. Frankencephalopathy (brain damage)
i. Unconsciousness
j. Focal neurological symptoms
k. permanent neurological and/or mental deficit

If you ask your pediatrician, she may tell you these are rare. Ask her to prove that statement. The problem with neurological damage, especially brain damage, is that there is often no black and white way of telling exactly where it came from. Brain damage often occurs insidiously over an extended period of time after the vaccine. The medical cartel's key argument is that after 48 hours, what ever happens is no longer the fault of a vaccine. This is the most horrendous of lies. When this level of toxicity is introduced into the blood, neurological damage can occur slowly over a period of years.

Many learning disabilities are mild forms of brain damage created by vaccine toxicity, and are not recognized until many years later while the child's school work becomes more challenging.

How about the MMR vaccine? Its' packet insert admits:

a. Moderate fever up to one month after injection (that's a bit more than 48 hours, wouldn't you say?)
b. High level fever up to 103 degrees.
c. Severe rash
d. Raised lesions at the injection site
e. Lymphadenopathy (swollen glands)
f. diarrhea
g. Convulsions
h. Optic neuritis and retinitis
i. Ocular palsies (eye paralysis)

In the 1970's when the Rubella vaccine was being tested, the federal department of *Health, Education and Welfare* wrote:

"As much as 26% of children receiving rubella vaccinations in national testing programs developed arthralgia (joint pain), and arthritis. Many had to seek medical attention and some were hospitalized, testing positive for rheumatic fever and rheumatoid arthritis."

In the next breath after admitting these symptoms "may" occur, they say it is unlikely. I can see why they do this. If you are able to suppress knowledge of actually how many thousands of children are hurt by vaccines, which is effectively done in the media, who would ever know the truth? Everyone affected believes they were the unlucky, rare bird of fate. A devious plan indeed. The packet inserts say that "no definite causal relationship has been established between these side effects and the vaccine." They can do this, because not everyone who gets a vaccine comes down with these symptoms. This is like believing cigarettes are not harmful because everyone who smokes does not develop cancer. Teams of lawyers hired by the medical cartel sit around for hours on the beach thinking this stuff up. I wonder if they *truthfully* vaccinate their kids? It is trickery and obfuscation to the greatest degree.

In late 1993, a TV program was aired called *"vaccine roulette."* It covered many issues concerning the dangers of the DPT vaccine. For example, in 1975 it took only 2 deaths of Japanese children following inoculations using the American DPT vaccine to ban its' use there forever. Strange as this may seem, this show in 1993 was simply a follow up program for a show on the dangers of DPT that was aired in 1982, which told the American public the exact same things. With all this threatening information out there, why was nothing done between the 11 years of these two programs? Why are American children still receiving the same DPT vaccine? From the show in 1982, called *"DPT, vaccine roulette:"*

"studies conducted by Sweden and West Germany found so much brain damage following DPT shots that neither government recommends this vaccine in any way. The only US government study done in over 50 years confirmed these European findings, but these findings have made no impact on American vaccine programs what so ever. The same US government study found that 1 in every 700 children had convulsions, or went into anaphylactic shock within 48 hours after their shot."

The AMA, head of propaganda for the medical cartel, responded to this show some months later by stating publicly that many people were now too scared to receive DPT shots, and therefore these respective disease rates were rapidly climbing. When this happens, the AMA always riles up a pressure cooker with politicians, stating they will be responsible for huge epidemics if they do not act to get the situation under control. Of course what this means to the AMA is forcing people to use their products and get vaccinated. Dr. Anthony Morris of the FDA (quoted in chapter one), actually went to Maryland and Wisconsin to examine for himself these AMA claims of increased disease rates. What he found, was that in Maryland only 5 of the 41 cases that were reported as diphtheria were actually confirmed. All 5 of these children had also been vaccinated with DPT! In Wisconsin, only 16 of the reported 43 cases of diphtheria were confirmed, and all but 2 of these confirmed 16 were vaccinated. So these vaccines are supposed to protect our children? I challenge any person with credentials to explain to me how this is done. Give me a call. We'll do lunch.

#3. *Vaccines are responsible for the decline of infectious diseases we have witnessed over the past 100 years.* This is an all out lie that has been pushed on the world through rewritten history books, as well as suppressed and altered data. We will discuss this further in Chapter 5, *Historical Chicanery.*

#4. Vaccines are the only way to prevent epidemic outbreaks. Vaccines can be proven today, to be the number one cause of anything close to an epidemic we may experience. I would question the validity of the **true nature** of any epidemic, from the bubonic plague (discussed in Chapter 7) to any present day manufactured one. Many so called epidemics have environmental origins that are conveniently overlooked by any author intent on placing blame to the germ theory. A good example of this occurred June of 1997 in Idaho. The contemporary news headline was, *"Low Vaccination Rates In Idaho Leading To Pertussis Outbreaks."* Despite this, here are the facts:

1. 86% of the cases of pertussis reported were in fully vaccinated people. This means the people had also received a Pertussis vaccine.
2. 14 % of these cases occurred in *partially* vaccinated people.
3. Only *ONE* person in this case was completely unvaccinated.

As a result of this newsbreak, the local health departments declared that 44% of the population of Idaho was at risk. They did not mention that all but one of them were already vaccinated however. Tricky! But it's done all the time folks. The CDC made sure they wrote in their report of this event that *"refusal of pertussis vaccine played no part in this outbreak."* You will notice, that they are always emphatic about this very point. You will very rarely see anything written by a government agency or drug company pointing blame at vaccines, despite the obvious facts starring them in the face.

Vaccination is simply a bad idea that has progressively, and aggressively gotten worse over time. I am certain that not all persons involved in their distribution and administration are *"evil."* There are many who are simply misguideded, which accounts for the bulk of society. But mark my word, *there is evil present here.* As is the case throughout history, it must be recognized and stopped by the caring actions of good people.

Injecting these poisons directly into the bloodstreams of our newborns is the hallmark of bad ideas gone worse; a prime example of how we are still existing under the auspices of an antiquated medical religion, which exists solely for its own gain as it preys upon innocent children as the demon behind the smiling mask. When are we going to stand up for ourselves and say, *THAT'S IT! NO MORE!* What is it going to take? Are we going to wait until half our population is autistic, mentally challenged or chronically ill? What is it going to take before we all band together to see the truth of what is really happening here?

Proportionally, a single vaccine given to a 6 pound newborn child in one day is the equivalent of giving a 180 pound person 30 vaccines on the same day. Would you like to experience what happens if someone were to give you 30 vaccines in one day? Include in this idea, the toxic effects of high levels of aluminum, mercury and formaldehyde contained in most vaccines, and the synergist toxicity could be increased to unknown astronomical levels. Further, it is very well known to science that infants do not produce significant levels of bile. Nor do they have adult renal capacity for several months after birth. Renal (Kidney) transport of bile is the major biochemical route by which Mercury is removed from the body, and infants can't do this at all well. They also do not possess the renal capacity to remove aluminum. Additionally, mercury is a well known inhibitor of kidney function and a potent neurotoxin. Considering all this, one can conclude through common sense that these "vaccines" are better suited for a tool of mass genocide. When are we going to wake up?

"There is no convincing scientific evidence that mass vaccination programs can be credited with eliminating any childhood disease. I urge you to reject all vaccinations for your child."

Robert Mendelsohn, MD

"As well consult a butcher on the value of vegetarianism as a doctor on the worth of vaccination."

George Bernard Shaw

"Vaccinations will one day go the way of bloodletting, and doctors of tomorrow will be shocked that without any good research showing any benefit, and much research showing harm, we continued using this bizarre 18th century medical practice of injecting viri, bacteria, toxins and other chemicals into our children well into the 21st century."

Tedd Koren, DC
vaccine researcher and author

Chapter Three

The Truth About Sudden Infant Death Syndrome and cancer

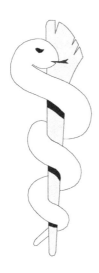

> *Part line #2* :   Sudden infant death syndrome is a still a mystery
> to medical science. More research is needed to find
> the pathogen, which is suspected to be a virus, or
> group of viruses that somehow overwhelm the
> infants immune system. After the virus is
> identified, a vaccine can be administered at some
> point during the first month of life.

"Crib death was so infrequent in pre-vaccination eras that it was not even mentioned in statistics. It only started to increase in the 1950's with mass vaccination programs."

Harris Coulter, Ph.D.

The AMA claims ignorance to what sudden infant death syndrome (SIDS) actually is. Valid research shows that it is nothing more than excess toxemia and brain damage the child receives as a result of vaccination.

A well known fact not discussed in the American press is that Japan increased their minimum vaccination age to 2 years old from 2 months old in 1975. Upon doing this, SIDS, spinal meningitis and many other related nervous system diseases virtually disappeared from the country. Japan then went from #17 in infant mortality to #1 in the world. Of course, children began to have all sorts of problems again beginning at age 2 when they received their vaccines.

Research also done by numerous Chiropractic organizations site Atlas subluxation to be a probable factor. Over 90% of SIDS cases are found to have this Atlas subluxation upon autopsy. The Atlas is the first neck vertebrae directly under the head.

Chiropractors believe that in addition to toxemia related to vaccines, modern hospital birthing procedures traumatize this delicate area of the spinal cord at the Atlas, called the brain stem. The Atlas subluxation, a mal-alignment of the vertebrae that places undue pressure on this area of the brain stem, can certainly interfere with proper respiratory and cardiac functions in an infant, even to the extent of shutting these systems down as the Atlas subluxation, which began at birth, becomes more chronic. Although the bulk of the medical profession hasn't a clue what to make of SIDS, they are very adept at telling you what is isn't. They are definitely not listening to the Chiropractors about Atlas subluxation, and they are emphatic that SIDS is not caused by vaccines. Can we trust them?

Reading the packet insert from the DPT vaccine from the Wyeth company:

"The occurrence of SIDS has been reported following the administration of DPT. The significance of these reports is unclear . . . ."

. . . . and remember, cigarettes don't cause cancer. The fact that SIDS is created by vaccine toxemia is only unclear to Wyeth.

Continuing on with the DPT packet insert:

"it should be kept in mind, that the three primary doses of DPT are usually administered to infants between the ages of 2 and 6 months, and that approximately 85% of all SIDS cases occur in the periods 1 to 6 months, with peak incidence at ages 2-4 months."

Are the significance of these reports still unclear to you? This is essentially an admission to guilt.

Older data from the CDC used to list that approximately 10,000 babies die per year from what is called "crib death," or SIDS. 85% of these cases occur within the second to forth month of life, and this just happens to coincide with the initial DPT and polio inoculations. This is not a coincidence.

Suppose you go into your pediatrician's office to get you child's DPT shot, and the doctor actually gave you a warning before hand. *"Mrs. Smith, let me first tell you that the assistant secretary of health testified before the US senate committee on May 3, 1985, that every year 35,000 children suffer some form of neurological damage, possibly even SIDS, as a result of receiving these vaccines. Okay, that's my disclaimer. Are you ready to give your child the shots?"*

When you call the CDC to obtain information on SIDS, they refer you to the propaganda center for SIDS, called the sudden infant death syndrome resource center. You can indeed receive a ton of resources from this resource center. I received information from them which states:

1. SIDS is the number one cause of death of infants between 1 month and one year, with peak incidence at 2 and 4 months.
2. SIDS is determined only after an autopsy, examination of the death scene, and a review of clinical history.
3. It is a recognized disorder, listed in the International Classification of diseases.
4. It is NOT caused by DPT vaccines or other vaccines.

How do professionals diagnose SIDS? According to the CDC:

"when an infant death is sudden and unexplained, investigators including medical examiners and coroners use the special expertise of forensic medicine. SIDS is no exception. Health professionals make use of 3 avenues of investigation. During the autopsy, a definitive diagnosis cannot be made without a through post mortem examination that fails to point to any other possible cause of death."

In other words, if the autopsy doesn't say the infant died from anything else, the diagnosis is SIDS. The medical profession uses SIDS as a garbage diagnosis when nothing else shows up, and this is a high crime, since the causes of SIDS are obvious and blatant. It should be reworded, that a mysterious infant death of this nature is presumed to be SIDS until further evidence proves otherwise.

Party line #3 :   We need more money for research to fight cancer
                     and chronic disease, which for some inconclusive
                     reason are reaching pandemic levels. A viral
                     culprit is suspected.

"Have we traded mumps and measles for cancer and leukemia in children?"

Robert Mendelshon, MD:
How to raise a healthy child in spite of your doctor:
1984

"The results of suppressing measles and other infectious diseases by vaccinations are cancer and other auto immune and chronic diseases."

V. Scheibner: Immunization:
The Medical assault on the immune system:
1993

"Measles vaccination in childhood was related to the following diseases in adult life: autoimmune diseases of bone and cartilage and certain tumors."

Lancet:
1985

In the 1950's during the polio vaccination campaigns, scientists learned that the polio vaccine administered to most children was contaminated with a highly carcinogenic monkey virus called SV40. The public was never notified and use of the vaccine was continued. By 1961 over 90% of school children received this carcinogenic virus from the vaccine, as over 100 million shots were given. As well, 62 studies from 30 world wide laboratories link the polio vaccine to brain tumors, bone cancers, lung lining cancers and leukemia, according to the American Association for Cancer Research in San Francisco (2002 study—*www.bmn.com*). The rates of all these cancers have gone up dramatically in the past 30 years, especially in children.

Cancer has been steadily on the rise in America amongst children since the onset of mandatory vaccination programs in the 1950's. Pediatric cancers are rising 1% per year since 1974 and are the leading cause of death in children after accidents. Leukemia and brain tumors are the most common childhood malignancies, having a 35% rise in pediatric brain cancer between 1973 and 1974, as reported by "Science" magazine in 1999.

Even though overwhelming evidence points to the obvious culprit, vaccines are not tested for their ability to cause cancer, mutations or developmental malformations. Nor are they tested to see if they will effect the child's reproductive system. These tests are routine for items like shampoo and cosmetics. But not for mandatory vaccines? Something is very wrong here, notwithstanding the obvious cancer connection to vaccines but also considering that over 25% of American couples are experiencing fertility problems since 1994.

"Cancer was practically unknown until smallpox vaccination began. I have never seen a case of cancer in a non-vaccinated person."
W.B. Clark, MD author

"I am convinced that some 80% of these cancer deaths are caused by smallpox vaccinations. These are well known to cause grave and permanent disease of the heart also."
Herbert Snow, MD: London Cancer Hospital

"I am convinced that the increase of cancer is due to vaccination."
Forbes Laurie, MD : Metro Cancer Hospital London

"The most frequent disposing condition for cancerous development is vaccination and re-vaccination."
Dennis Turnbull, MD Cancer researcher

Regarding the nature of chronic and fatal disease related to vaccine abuse, one must first understand the nature of a virus. So what is a virus? Many in the natural healing community don't even believe they exist; not naturally anyway. Being that they don't eat, excrete, breathe, move freely or reproduce, viruses do not fit the criteria for organic life as we know it. In fact, *no one* has ever seen a live virus. They are so small, they can only be viewed under intense magnification which requires specially prepared dead tissue. Let's say some pharmaceutical company grants a large sum of money to a University to find the polio viruses we spoke of in the last chapter. As you know, the monkey's kidney is injected with poisons until it becomes very sick. A researcher can culture some of that monkey's kidney tissue to look for the viruses, and there you have it! Lo and behold, every time the researcher cultures that sick monkey's kidney, viruses are found suspected to cause polio. But what is the researcher really looking at?

It is a known fact that toxemia of any body tissue causes the cell membranes to break down. The cells of any disease tissue actually lyce, or explode. When they do, the cell membranes shatter much like your car windshield would if you got into a car accident. They shatter, and tiny pieces fall all over the place quickly. Viruses are little pieces of cell membrane with genetic material inside. Inside each Human cell, there is a nucleus which contains genetic material called DNA (deoxyribo nucleic acid). This nucleus has a nuclear membrane which is practically identical to the cell membrane. There is also a roadway to the nucleus of each Human cell called the endoplasmic reticulum. It has Ribosome's connected to it, and Ribosome's also contain genetic material called RNA (ribo nucleic acid). This endoplasmic reticulum is also made of cellular membrane material. Each Human cell is actually a swimming pool with these organelles contained in a watery mixture called Cytoplasm. Cytoplasm also contains the genetic material RNA. So as you can see, there is no shortage of genetic material in any Human cell. In toxemia, when the cell bursts due to lysis, there is an abundance of cellular membrane material containing the sticky proteins of DNA and RNA now floating in the fluid between the other living cells, called the interstitial fluid. This process is similar to your car windshield bursting with one of those fine line radio antennas inside it. Pieces of the antennae will be found in many of the shattered pieces of windshield. Similarly, it is normal to find tiny pieces of cell membrane with DNA or RNA inside it, or stuck to it, in a sick person. There is a lot of cell lysis due to their levels of toxemia. This is what many lab technicians, MD's and researchers are looking at under high magnification when looking for "viruses." They have simply given a name to a phenomena of cellular toxemia, calling it a "virus" and placing on it as much blame as they can.

This idea of a "viral organism" is not one backed by any real scientific fact, since viruses aren't even alive! Can a virus enter a normal, healthy Human cell and start creating havoc within a person? Yes, I still believe they can, but this happens much like a rock being hauled at your car windshield while driving. These dead fragments of cellular membrane with genetic material either caught inside of it or stuck to it, create havoc in an otherwise healthy cell since they are invaders, proteinaceous and genetic in nature. This invasion can create an overload of stress to the cell, but the invasion is not coming from any kind of invading *"organism."* It is coming from these scattered pieces of junk, or cellular debris which are abundant in all toxic people. However, one must also realize that any so called virus that can invade a cell can also be manufactured purposely to do so. Governments from many countries, especially the United States, have run wild with this viral theory, working on creating a microscopic monster since WWII. The goal is the ultimate weapon for germ warfare. Manufactured, or man made genetic material, can certainly be created as a lethal weapon. Genes from various sources that don't belong together can be spliced into a killer strand of DNA or RNA. Wrap this genetic material in a cell membrane carrier vehicle and you have your ultimate weapon. This genetic material is so toxic that it causes cells to explode the moment it crosses the cell membrane.

When injected, on purpose, in high concentrations into the blood, these free floating RNA and DNA genetic molecules float into the cell and through the nuclear membrane. Within the nucleus they can cause severe disruptions to the cells ability to divide normally, or recreate itself, as cells do millions of times per day. God created a perfect reproducing organism without flaws. This genetic material interferes with that very principle. When the cell cannot reproduce normally, it is damaged, and acts to produce a damaged organism. This can even cause the cell to divide wildly, with toxic imperfections and out of control, which is the fundamental basis of cancer.

Live and attenuated viral vaccines provide you with this highly toxic genetic material. It has always floored me, that parents give these shots to their children without a single question as to the nature of their contents. What is there to stop a government or military organization from placing experimental genetic material into vaccines, to control select populations at will? Do you really believe these organizations are beyond that type of action? By administering genetic fragments into the blood, cancer and mutations are far more likely than increased resistance to disease. Since childhood cancer is now the leading cause of childhood disease death, one should take these facts very seriously. These genetic fragments cause the cell to divide abnormally, and this again, is the fundamental basis of all cancers known to plague Humankind.

In 1976, Dr. Robert Simpson of Rutgers University was addressing science writers at a seminar of the American Cancer Society. He said:

> "... immunization programs against flu, measles, mumps, polio and so forth may actually be seeding Humans with RNA to form latent proviruses in cells throughout the body. These latent proviruses are molecules in search of creating disease, including rheumatoid arthritis, multiple sclerosis, lupus, Parkinson's disease and cancer ..."

In his book, *"The Case Against Immunizations,"* Richard Moskowitz, MD writes:

> "... these genetic particles attach their own genetic material as an extra particle or episome to the chromosome of the host cell,

and replicate along with it. This allows the host cell to continue its' own normal functions for the most part, but it places upon it additional instructions for the synthesis of viral proteins. This presence of antigenic material in the host cell cannot fail to produce auto immune phenomena, such as herpes, shingles, warts, tumors both benign and malignant, and diseases of the central nervous system such as various forms of paralysis and inflammation of the brain . . ."

As a reminder, AIDS, lupus, multiple sclerosis, rheumatoid arthritis and cancer are all autoimmune diseases. Fact of the matter is, the vaccination campaigns that have been hoisted upon the American public over the past 50 years are directly responsible for the astronomical increases in cancer we are seeing today. Diet and environmental toxins are also a piece of the cancer puzzle, but they shy next to this vaccination component.

The late Dr. Robert Bell had quite a few credentials to his name. Cancer specialist of the British Medical Hospital, president of the *medical association for the reduction and prevention of cancer*, Vice President of the *International Society of Cancer Research,* and member of the *American Society of Progressive Physicians*. He simply had this to say in 1982. Short and not so sweet:

" . . . the chief, if not sole cause of the monstrous increase in cancer has been vaccinations . . ."

Research over the past 50 years on the correlation between cancer and vaccinations is difficult, if not impossible to find. The CDC and AMA have made sure of this. You will also be hard pressed to find a case of cancer in an unvaccinated person, especially an unvaccinated child. This research and thought never makes its' way into the main stream for very good reasons. Primarily, it's really bad for business. Can you imagine a media story about an unvaccinated child that is super healthy? This is the AMA's worst nightmare. The reader should start thinking CDC = NIH = AMA =

FDA = Law makers = Pharmaceutical company. They are all part of the same club organization rendering huge profits from the business of keeping people very sick and diseased. Once you have a stable population of sick people constantly using your services, you can make further profits on *"taking care"* of them. This is a crime only the devil could have masterminded. You must wake up to the fact, or at least begin to consider, that all those who follow it are either demons themselves, or victims of mass brainwashing.

Dr. K. Morrison, formally professor of chemistry and toxicology at the National University of Washington, member of the medical council and an examiner in the college of physicians and surgeons in Canada, said in 1984:

"... two well known causes of cancer are 1. Nicotine, and 2. Vaccinations. Vaccines are certainly the most prolific cause of internal and external cancer. The vaccine virus poisons the lymphatic system, impairs its function and lays the foundation for internal cancer, from which there has not been any successful medical treatment to date ..."

From *"The poison needle,"* by Elanor Mcbean, Dr. Charles E. Paser of Boston University wrote in 1989:

"... I have been a regular practitioner of medicine in Boston for 33 years. I have studied the question of vaccinations conscientiously for 45 years. As for vaccinations as a preventative of disease, there is not a scrap of evidence in its' favor. Injection of virus into the pure blood stream of the people does not prevent disease. Rather, it tends to increase epidemic and make the disease it is attempting to annihilate more deadly. Of this we have indisputable proof. In America, cancer mortality has increased from 9 cases per 100,000 to 80 cases per 100,000, or a 900% increase over the last 50 years. No conceivable thing could have caused this but the universal blood poisoning now existing in the form of vaccinations ..."

By the time children in America reach the age of 14, they receive anywhere from 20 to 30 separate vaccinations. The pharmaceutical companies and the government want you to receive more as well! According to them, your body is not clean enough unless you have these vaccines, and you are a threat to society. Each time you receive one of these vaccines, the risk of long term damage to your body increases, and toxins accumulate to create chronic disease. The American Cancer Society tells us that the leading killer disease in children before the age of 14, is cancer. Statistically, if a person acquires a fatal cancer, death will occur within 5 years ***with medical treatment.*** If a person does not seek any kind of treatment, death occurs within an average of 12 years. Is this merely a coincidence? Any novice crime investigator would tell you no.

Chapter Four

Who's afraid of the big bad FLU?

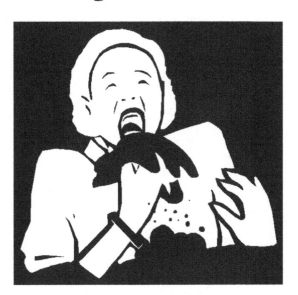

Party Line #4:	The multitudes of bacterial and viral strains that cause the common cold and flu are staggering. Each year there are endless new varieties, since these micro-organisms are able to mutate and adapt so rapidly. This has been the ongoing dilemma with finding an all encompassing cure for the common cold and flu, and precisely why flu shots are needed every year. Before each "flu Season," which begins with the onset of the cold weather, our brilliant medical researchers work diligently to isolate the new strains so that vaccines can be provided for the public before the season begins. Thus, research has shown that flu vaccines have greatly decreased the incidence of flu in North America.

What a load of malarkey! The medical cartel, using the CDC's political influence, has successfully developed this elaborate, and quite profitable *witch hunt* called the *"Flu Season."* Part of the reason they are able to do this; a huge part that is, has to deal with the psychological state of our nation in regards to accepting responsibility for their own health, and the creation of their own illness. It is so much easier for a people, brainwashed into denial, to accept that they have become invaded by some new microbe that systematically has the power to bring them down. This is precisely why people go running for flu shots each year before the holidays. For all intents and purposes, the wise, educated individual should at least realize the high level of chicanery involved in the language of "cold and flu seasons."

What the medical cartel has capitalized as "cold" and "flu" are nothing more than the bodies intent, sometimes extreme, to detoxify. Let's go over some of the myths of this "cold and flu season:"

1. *It's cold outside! The body's resistance to germs is lower in cold weather, which is why people primarily get sick when the weather changes to cold.*

Actually, part of this is true. The Human body is placed under stress during periods of cold weather, and it is important to keep from becoming too chilled while outside. This is especially important for young children and infants. However, cold or warm has nothing to do with resistance to so called "germs." We will discuss this further when we fully take apart the germ theory. For now, just understand that this notion of contagion becoming more communicable in cold weather has no basis in rational science. What does become lower however in cold weather, is your body's ability to maintain a high threshold for toxicity. When this occurs, you start coughing up, spitting up, and ejecting mucous from every orifice the body can eject accumulated poison from.

2. *Beware the "Strept Throat" boggie man's a comin!*

Strept throat cultures are the biggest scam since pink lemonade. Kids get sore throats. Parents haul them into the pediatrician in fear. The doctor gets a throat culture and gives you a call the next day saying they found *streptococcus*. Your kid then goes on antibiotics for Strept throat, gets better in some weeks and everyone lives happily ever after. Only, if you repeat this exact same scenario, save the sore throat or any thought of illness, you may still have a positive culture for streptococcus! In other words, these streptococcus are there whether or not you get the diagnosis of strept throat. These cultures, and the diagnosis, are virtually meaningless. Now repeat the same scenario with a suspected illness, and take out the antibiotics. The recovery time for your child will most likely be shorter, if not the same. Antibiotics should rarely be taken by anyone, especially children. They are highly toxic to children, and should only be given to anyone during a life threatening crisis where detoxification runs out of control.

Parents should understand that during the cold weather months, children and adults will get sore throats primarily due to dry, cold weather; and dry, warm forced air indoor heating environments. These two things dry up the otherwise moist mucous membranes of the nasal and throat passages (called the nasopharynx), causing them to crack just enough to enhance irritation. The microbes found around these cracked and dry throat membranes are simply there doing the job God created them to do; eating up toxic waste build up. The microbes' metabolism of your body's garbage, now found in these cracked and dry throat membranes, are what cause the sore throat feeling. The culprit however, is not the microbe. It is the level of toxicity you have in your own blood stream that now has the chance to ooze out.

3. *Influenza epidemics peak mysteriously at the same time of year throughout the U.S., 4 to 6 weeks after January 1. It is not known what creates these elevations, but they may be due to delayed reporting following the Christmas and New Years holidays.*

Well, these united cycles of illness called "influenza" are very related to the holidays, but they have nothing to do with germs or delayed reporting. We all know what happens around the holidays. Thanksgiving rolls around the third Thursday of November to begin the whole show. Americans eat a lot. A lot of meat. A lot of booze. Coffee. Tea. White sugar products. White flour products. Stress of being around family members we would only agree to be around because of the holidays. We may well survive this assault of multiple stress, just in time for Christmas shopping! Then all of the above begins once again. Then we have our New Years celebration. Then all of the above begins once more. Then your body finally has enough of all this, and screams, *"I'M NOT GOING TO TAKE THIS ANYMORE!"* and you get sick! But are you really "sick," in the full sense of the word? No, you're not. In fact, you are more healthy than the person who cannot produce symptoms of detoxification anymore because the body's vitality has been beaten down.

This is the real story of the CDC's *mysterious* flu epidemic, that arises annually for 6 weeks around the holidays. The CDC will tell you that these supposed flus are contagious, and it is wise to get your vaccine. What a scam! Mostly everyone is detoxifying without understanding why, and the medical cartel seizes the moment for profit with its' propaganda on a naive and foolish public. There have been little, if any, double blind studies completed by the pharmaceutical companies comparing people who take their medications (antibiotics, over the counter cold and flu remedies and the like) with people who do absolutely nothing but rest and drink more water. They absolutely refuse to complete *any double blind* studies on the effectiveness of flu vaccinated people with the unvaccinated population. Why is this so? Because they already know what the results would be. Sickness in the vaccinated population is equal to, and most likely greater than, sickness in the unvaccinated. If this were true of any other company you or I began, we would be shut down immediately by the FDA and other federal agencies. But the medical cartel gets to run amok without any supporting evidence of effectiveness.

For those of you who need a review, a double blind study involving the effectiveness of any given vaccine would commence as follows. A group of people to study would all be *told* they were receiving a certain vaccine, however, only a certain select number out of the group would actually receive the vaccine, and the rest would receive water. The people administering the shots, as well as the people collecting the data after the shots were given, would also not know which shots were the actual vaccines, and which shots were simply water. Only a select few researchers would have this information. There would also be a *control* group of people who received no shots. These three distinct groups would then be studied over the course of a year or more. What would the result be? No one knows, because the drug companies who make the shots refuse to commence such a project in a truly scientific manner, using a third party research company to complete the study to ensure reliability of the collected data.

I can tell you from my own personal research without a doubt, that the incidence of cold or flu in each group would come out equal, probably with the real vaccinated group showing more illness in general than the other two groups. This would once and for all prove that vaccines are a scam, but the drug companies are totally and unequivocally made unaccountable for the thousands of lives they damage annually through their methods and medications. No one in government is pushing for a study such as this one, and for good reason. The medical cartel forbids it. They have become their own form of government within our government, and in some areas control our lives more than any other form of government we have ever seen. Watch out for this medical profession and cartel; they aim to control more of your life as each year passes.

Even the World Health Organization has conceded that the most common protection against infectious diseases is an adequate diet. If this is the case, why isn't the medical profession, with all its' advertising prowess, aiming people toward taking better care of themselves by eating better? The answer is simple. There's no profit in empowering people to be healthy, and keep themselves that way. They make it perfectly clear that they will continue to act as the real drug pushers of our society, pushing their massive vaccine campaigns through government, assuring a compliant and available public for profit.

It is vital to have a clear understanding of the true nature of cold and flu, especially if you are a parent. These conditions are, in a sense, a *"contagious"* process of detoxification and elimination. Even the *chicken pox*, thought to be contagious, is simply a natural process of immune system development that most children need to experience. I have recommended the homeopathic remedy *Rhus Toxicodendron* in my practice for many years, and have never seen a case of chicken pox it did not help the child process through in 48 hours or less, without scarring!

Cold weather does precipitate colds and flus, not due to any more virulent germ of the cold weather, but more from the emotional and physical stress we experience during the cold weather months. Forced air, dry and enclosed heating environments severely dry the outer skin, as well as the inner. The inner linings of the nose, pharynx, throat, larynx and bronchial tubes are called *mucous membranes,* because they are naturally lined with a healthy layer of moist fluid. This layer is drastically reduced in forced air, non moist indoor heating environments, and thus is prone to becoming torn and chaffed (in other words, a sore throat). Toxins in the blood now come to the surface, the natural saprophytic (garbage eating) qualities of the bacteria ever present in these areas goes to work, they start to metabolize and excrete as they work, and you now have what the medical profession calls a full blown cold or flu. All other lung diagnoses, such as bronchitis, pneumonia and the like follow the same rule of thumb here of a respiratory system detoxification process. With concern to detoxification, the lungs and respiratory system in general are a huge outlet for toxicity, and when it is vital the body uses this avenue of toxic release quite often.

What a person thinks of as catching a contagious cold or flu, can also be a recent reaction to an environmental toxin. Chlorine vapors from indoor hot tubs and pools greatly irritate the respiratory linings, especially in the winter. Chlorine vapors, when breathed in for an extended period of time actually burn the respiratory mucous membranes. The body then creates these symptoms to spit out the toxic mix of chlorine infested, dead cellular material. Leaf blowing without a proper mask kicks up an array of junk that also gets lodged in the respiratory tract. Everything from mold spores to environmental toxins can be inhaled for an extended period of blowing leaves around your yard. Spending hours cleaning out a dusty, murky crawl space can do the same. There are many similar examples of daily life that can create this scenario.

Many of my patients complain over the years that they have no choice but to take antibiotics, for if they don't the cold or flu process will consume them for weeks, possibly even months. They give antibiotics to their children as prescribed by their medical doctor, out of fear of them getting worse and possibly harmed further. I have yet to see a single case of cold or flu, in either my personal or professional life, that does any better with a prescription of antibiotics. I suggest my patients administer homeopathic remedies for cold and flu symptoms, and these work far better than antibiotics could ever dream of working. Homeopathy is also non-toxic, whereas antibiotics are highly toxic to a child's developing bone marrow.

However, even with homeopathy, a person must realize that the purpose of the cold or flu is *detoxification.* Whatever is being spit out of the body, through whatever orifice, needs to be spit out. Anything you take or give to alleviate or shut down symptoms is going to shut down this healing process and keep the toxicity inside you. Then your body will have to develop other symptoms at some time down the road in order to compensate. An exception to this are some schools of Naturopathy and Homeopathy which give remedies solely to enhance the healing process, and not target the elimination of symptoms. You can never win at the symptom suppression game, because as long as you are living and vital, your body will attempt to do its' job of making you as pure as possible.

There is a practical argument regarding cold and flu that, being a parent myself, I have to agree with. How much is enough? At what point does a parent have to draw the line and say, "this is all the detoxification I can take for one day!" I do feel that this line has to be drawn, regarding the parents' or the child's symptoms. Outside of a life threatening situation, I would never give a child antibiotics. Homeopathy for children is wonderful and for the most part, non-invasive. Parents should consider the same guidelines regarding antibiotics for themselves, simply due to the liver toxic nature of such drugs. Homeopathy is the best choice for an ailing, busy parent on the run, and I have yet to meet a good parent who was not busy and on the run taking care of their children.

Cough suppressants are also necessary *at times* when either the parents' or child's coughing becomes too severe. The lungs build up a myriad of dirt and pollution from the outside. From the indoor, artificially heated world, the lungs receive a myriad of items floating around in the air, like dead skin cells with dust mites on them, mold and fungus spores, and vaporized chemicals amongst the most irritating of things. During a cold or flu detoxification process, these things mix with thick mucus. The body does this to expectorate these toxins out of the lungs once and for all. These mentioned toxins, mixed with the microbes feasting on them, are what give the mucus its' green and yellow colors. Mucus can also be red and orange in color when mixed with blood due to the cracking of the dry, inner mucus membranes of the respiratory system. Each winter my patients complain that their cough worsens at night, at times to the point where they feel they may need a hospital. The coughing goes on and on and on at night, usually waking them up about an hour or so after they have fallen asleep. Coughing to expectorate lung toxicity is normally going to be more active at night. This coughing, in contrast to popular medical belief, is not contagious. But it will keep a person up all night and leave him exhausted in the morning. This is because as you sleep, your body obtains more vitality to spit this garbage out of you than it has when you are busy doing many things during the day.

By all means, if you have to take a Homeopathic cough suppressant (there are many good ones on the market), or worse yet, a nationally advertised popular brand, do so if the release process is consuming your time to sleep. Otherwise the next day you won't be able to do anything if you have an important meeting, have to be at work or need to take care of children. Understand however, that this action has its' consequences. You will get another batch of symptoms at sometime down the road, possibly even worse than you have now. The only way to totally end this cold and flu cycle is to take more responsibility for your body's level of ongoing toxicity. When you take the right steps to *"clean out,"* colds and flus will be a thing of the past. Of course, if you have these symptoms and are able to stay at home for some days to let them run their course, then it is best you cough all night and sleep all day. Here are my most beneficial suggestions regarding colds and flus. If you follow them to the letter, you will eliminate these things from your life forever:

1. **Go on two 7 day fasts.** One in the spring and one in the summer. This is a time you have to yourself where you can just lay around and drink water. You will eat nothing for this time period. Afterwards, break your fast with fresh fruit and raw vegetables for two days. If you can't do 7 days, try 3 or 4 days minimum. Supervision from a natural doctor can be beneficial with this process.

2. **Fasting is best, but if you feel you just can't do that, at least clean up your diet to be more wholesome.** Eat only organic meats and vegetables, and be sure to have a "raw" portion with each meal, usually raw vegetables. *Eat fruit only by itself!* Have a fruit breakfast every morning, and eat only fruit up until noon. Regulate your caffeine drinks to one or two cups *per week*, especially during the cold weather. Decaffeinated drinks are fine. Caffeine is a respiratory irritant, and has been known to cause uncontrollable fits of coughing if you are already going through a detoxification process.

3. **Give up dairy products for good, especially milk and cheese.** Regardless of what you've been told, you get no calcium, or otherwise good nutrition from these products. Cow milk, with its' huge protein molecules and different sugars, is made for baby cows, not humans. The human metabolic systems and body temperature are very different from the cow, which makes cow milk virtually indigestible, and thus useless.

4. **Drink plenty of high quality, thin drinking water.** One of the finest products on the market today is called PENTA, and can be purchased at most health food stores by the case and single bottle. This is an ultra thin water that gets in and out of the body cells very quickly, creating a very effective, non bloating cleanse. Visit *www.hydrateforlife.com,* or *www.pentawater.com.*

5. **Be responsible with the obvious.** Smoking of any kind, recreational drugs and alcohol build up toxicity in your body like nothing else can.

6. **Cleanse your home of mold, fungus and spores.** Ventilation and heating companies can help you do this, but these things are abundant in and under your old carpeting as well.

7. **Purchase an Ozone and Ionic generating air purifier to oxidize dead skill cells and molds in your indoor breathing environment.** This will eliminate the food supply of dust mites, and they will begin to die off. The ozone also oxidizes mold and fungus in some portions of your home's carpeting.

Chapter Five

9-11 terrorism paranoia and a pharmaceutical company's dream come true.

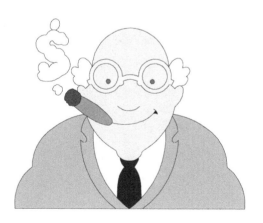

The world is certainly a different place after 9-11, and the truth seeker needs to know it is due to the carefully orchestrated, stealthily planned events which happened on that terrible day. 9-11 was the beginning of the "end game" for complete global control which will eventually leave the Illuminati as emperors if the people do not wake up soon, and take a firm stand against the loss of liberty and the rise of tyranny from those who would "protect" us. I have researched the events of 9-11 extensively since that day, and where this text is not designed for such a discussion, I wholeheartedly encourage the reader to discover the facts using the following references.

9/11: The Great Illusion; George Humphrey: PO Box
    5772, Austin TX 78763
www.fearorlove.com

Painful Questions, Eric Hufschmid: 1-800-258-7599
http://hiddenmysteries.com

Alice and Wonderland and the World Trade Center Disaster,
    David Icke 1-800-444-2524
www.davidicke.net

9-11, Descent into Tyranny, Alex Jones, 1-888-253-3139
http://www.infowars.com

As well, I will use this noun, *"Illuminati,"* frequently throughout the text. Who are the people within this organized crime tribe? The

Illuminati are a well organized, highly influential and extremely wealthy (and thus powerful) group of essentially one thousand or so people, consisting of several interbreeding blood line families. These families have been behind the scenes controlling politics, war and economies for hundreds of years. Their primary agenda is to control the lives of every human being on the planet in as many ways as you can imagine, with themselves as the undisclosed world dictators. They are very, very close to accomplishing this task.

A complete understanding of the Illuminati requires a bit of research; so much more than can be offered in this text. For the most complete and up to date information on them, read **David Icke's** magnificent book, *"The Biggest Secret,"* available on-line and at most book stores for around $25.

"At what point then, is the approach of danger to be expected? I answer, if it ever reaches us, it must bring up amongst us. It can not come from abroad. If destruction be out lot, we must ourselves be it's author and finisher."
President Abraham Lincoln, 1860

The orchestrations of 9-11-01 were vitally necessary for the power elite's agenda of progressive world domination. Those Warren-commission-esk baby stories fed to the American people since 9-11 are a typical form of the manipulative propaganda portrayed throughout history by warmongers; i.e., those whose make money and gain power from the activities of war, no matter the final outcome. *It was physically impossible by the laws of nature* for those buildings to come down as fast as they did through the "pancake" method explained. The heat produced from the engine fuel explosions could not possibly have created the infernal environment to melt the steal frames, which would require a minimum of 2,700 degrees F. Jet fuel from airlines burns no higher than 1,800 degrees F in the best of conditions. Considering that much of the heat escaped outside the building, this event alone could not bring the buildings down. The planes crashing into the buildings were the magician's diversion.

Several days after 9-11 aerial photographs and heat readings were taken by NASA. Five days after the event, some areas at "ground zero" were measuring greater than 1,300 degrees F. They want you to believe that two kamikaze airliners created all this heat, five days after the fact? Sure, and next year the Easter bunny will go door to door delivering American flags on the forth of July. Why not? Rah Rah Rah! Go America! What a marvelous country! Neither tons of jet fuel, nor a compression demolition have the potential to create this type of heat, much less maintaining it for five days!

Without any proof whatsoever of "who really done it", convenient judgments were formed, culprits were condemned, and a military take over of a portion of the world much sought after for it's wealth in commerce began. Many more people were killed from the initial phases of this takeover than in the 9-11 disaster, most of them old men, women and children (European and India press reported a range of 5,500 to 25,000 causalities). We have all been duped into believing, once again, that the evil bad guys need to be rounded up and eliminated to ensure "freedom and world peace" . . . . or as they say, a "new world order." The trick that has been played on society so successfully throughout history by the power elite, is to create a massive cultural subconscious of *primal fear.* Fear takes us out of our space of reason and compassion, and destroys our intellectual process, rendering us preoccupied with survival mode. Those who do not use their God given power of objective intellectual reasoning are controlled by the vagrancies of an undisciplined mind, and are at the whim of whatever propaganda is convenient to be pushed on them.

An interesting fact to always remember is this; in the week just before 9-11, there was an increase of 1200% in trading activity of orders going "short" on the stocks of American and United Airlines. This was reported by the Chicago Securities Exchange. As many of you know, when an investor goes short he expects the stock to decrease in value, and thus makes a lot of money on the company's demise. The highest percentage of this activity (reported by the NY Times & Wall Street Journal) came from Deutche Bank/ AB Brown. To date, there has been no investigation into how this company had foreknowledge of these 9-11 associated airlines. I suppose Martha Stewart is far more dangerous to society than this wealthy group of robber barons with foreknowledge of the worst terrorist attack in human history.

The bulk of society is easily duped in this way; easily moved by the self destructive energies of hate, revenge, anger, confusion, and fear. The Illuminati know this aspect of human psychology very well, and have been using it as a measure of control, passed down by teaching their generations of club members throughout the centuries.

Just how does all this fit in with the main topic of this book; i.e., "germs" and medical frauds? The connection to consider is the one the "state" will enforce on you and your children to be medicated for the good of society, or indefinitely quarantined. Plans for this are in the works.

So then, how did all this madness, centered around a global paranoia of these ghosts called "*germs*" begin? What are the deeper connections to 9-11? Like all other modes of oppression we so prevalently experience on our planet today, the groundwork was laid stealthily, cautiously and with precision over the past two centuries. The master plan of the Illuminati; those who I call *Club Conspiracy;* that 1.5% of the planet's population who control the flow of banking currency and most of the worlds corporations and industry, have sought to control all life on Earth for a very long time. It's not enough that they control, either directly or indirectly, the flow of money and property in all countries, severely polarizing the planet into a classic Marxist dream of privileged and proletariat. In order to accomplish their *end game,* 9-11 was skillfully engineered with all the mysterious "holes" of a dead Kennedy conspiracy (Jack, Bobby, and John Jr.). Their ultimate master plan for a totalitarian rule requires full control of your biological property as well; i.e., your body and the bodies off all your children. They are accomplishing this by one of three venues;

1. Concealing the truth about the mastery of your magnificent human organism with germ theory ghost stories, making

you psychologically dependant. This is accomplished primarily through the control of medical and healing arts educational curriculum and practice, and of course, the media.

2. Encouraging a lifestyle of poor health choices and bad habits. This leads down a road to inevitable sickness and dis-ease of the body. The final bad choice in this scenario is depending on the pharmaceutical and medical professions to get well.

3. Adherence to their germ theory religion, and the total acceptance of all their toxic products to the call of mandatory exclusion of all other natural remedies for, *"the good of the state,"* by enforcement through the corrupt UNITED STATES judicial system.

To the Illuminati who own and run the medical and pharmaceutical cartels, you are nothing but a piece of biological property needing to be controlled. They are presently after your body and the bodies of your children. Are you going to hand them over willingly? Are you going to volunteer? You need to speak up now while you still have a choice. Since 9-11, the pharmaceutical and medical cartels are actively, and fervently pushing with an unyielding passion to become the next branch of "government." They want to enforce treatment of anyone they wish, and for whatever reason at their whim, especially your children.

Buck the "system" too much and happen to get arrested for "disorderly conduct?" They want the legal rights to "treat" you with drugs and other "therapies" while incarcerated to become a "better citizen."

"What!? You don't want to get vaccinated!? You refuse to have your children vaccinated!? We really encourage you to "volunteer" to get your shots. Don't be foolish! There is danger in the form of noxious germs all around you! What kind of a parent are you!?" The next thing you know as a result of this monologue, the medical cartel will have the power to take your children out of your home and forcefully vaccinate them. If you do not "volunteer," you will spend an indefinite period of time in a state "quarantine" facility run by the local health department and DCF. They will have complete power to keep you there until you comply like a good pet and get your shots.

Does your child disrupt the class, and show that he may need to learn in a different way than is pushed upon most kids in our average "sheeple" public school mentality? They want the legal right to take your child from your home and "treat" him in a specialized institution with drugs and other "therapies," until he shows more compliance. Or perhaps your child has developed cancer from the toxic chemicals her weakened body has been trying to fight as a result of receiving 74 medical vaccines before the age of 6. You want to say, "that's enough!" But you can't. They want, and in some cases feel they already have, the legal right to force chemotherapy, radiation and other toxic "treatments" on your child against your will. Since 1980 there have been several cases where the judicial system has ordered toxic medical treatments for children totally overriding the will of the parents. In a few of these cases the parents left the state, were eventually abducted by law enforcement officials and arrested for kidnapping! Be sure to see our *REMEDIES* section for the forms and filings on re-owning yourself and your children through UCC-1 filings and common law copyrights.

When viewed objectively from a historical prospective, one can see that the events of 9-11 were the classic set up using the Hegelian Principal. Georg Wilhelm Hegel (1770-1831) was a German philosopher who is today considered one of the most influential thinkers in modern times. Hegel's articulation and teaching concerning successive phases in the consciousness and awareness of man is still part of the bedrock of philosophical teaching. He is known for the theorem: Thesis, Antithesis and Synthesis. A simplified English translation is: Problem, Reaction, and Solution. For hundreds of years the Illuminati have used the Hegelian process to further their cause; they secretly create a problem, the general population reacts with fear, and the solution is to transfer power to those who originally created the problem. This method is tried and true, however effective and diabolical.

Here are some historical events where the Hegelian process was used as explained, besides of course 9-11:

1. Bombing plans for Pearl Harbor was known months in advance by Roosevelt's agents. Information was never given to the naval base commander because he wanted a reason to enter into WWII, since at the time Americans were overwhelmingly opposed to getting involved in either the European or Asian conflicts.
2. Hitler burned down the Reichstag building (German Capitol) and blamed it on his opponents. Within days he arrested and executed many of his political adversaries.
3. After the Alfred P. Murrah building was bombed in Oklahoma, Clinton and his gang pushed the "Anti-Terrorist" legislation through congress within days. This legislation, especially in conjunction with "Patriot" acts I and II, tears the united states constitution and the bill of rights to shreds.

As is the present case with 9-11, the ridiculously misnamed "Patriot" Acts I and II are only the beginning. Now the federal government has the ability to arrest anyone they want at any time on a subjective suspicion of "terrorism," and incarcerate them without a trial indefinitely. Now the medical cartel wants their piece of the pie; i.e., your body. They want the rights to do whatever they want to do with it for the good of "public health," and the prevention of "terrorism." If *we the people* are not vigilant in our quest for freedom, they will gain the authority to inject us and our children with medical chemicals on a regular basis, without us being able to do anything about it. The orchestrations for such plans are already drawn up by Center for Disease Control officials, just waiting for the right climate to pounce upon the American people.

It is a well-known fact that the policy makers of the Center for Disease Control (the CDC) have intimate ties to pharmaceutical companies and lawmakers. Many decision makers at the CDC hold shares in the pharmaceutical companies, which make the vaccines they push on lawmakers. Since the panic, which has been created by 9-11, the CDC now realizes they have a stronger hold on such lawmakers, and thus your life. In effect, being that there is a declared time of crisis in our country, the CDC has the power to forcefully medicate you with the very vaccines they profit from. The vaccines that have been proven to kill and maim thousands of GI's and children every year.

What a marvelous marketing tool! Can you imagine how wealthy you would become if the government forced everyone AT GUNPOINT to use a product you have invented?! You would be rich beyond your wildest dreams, and that is exactly what the corrupt CDC aims to do by their now relentless pressuring of state and federal lawmakers to pass "*Public Health Emergency*" statutes (laws) that would require EVERYONE to be vaccinated at the push of a button.

Think this is all too far fetched? Well then, consider this headline from **USA Today**;

"Smallpox Fear Grips Nation" . . . . CDC Orders 100 Million-Dose Vaccine Stockpile" . . . . Untested Vaccine Will Be Mandatory During Public Health Emergencies" . . . . State Militia May be Mobilized to Enforce Vaccination Policies" . . . .

What a bizarre headline! Isn't it curious in this time of post 9-11 paranoia we are experiencing, that state militias have nothing better to do than be available to mobilize people into lines like cattle to receive shots?!

Let me get straight to the point here without mincing words to keep you comfortable; the pharmaceutical companies, CDC, and lawmakers which support them could give a rats ass if you die from smallpox. To them, you are an expendable resource; a *thing* to be used to gain more power through more cash. Believe me, you will soon realize that they will take full advantage of this time of crisis and pull every string they have now to bring these forced vaccination laws into effect.

Here's something I'll bet you did not know; in the late 70's when that peanut farmer we had for a president sold out to the tune of big government, he signed into effect FEMA, which stands for the Federal Emergency Management Act. You saw these guys walking all around the Trade Center ruins with FEMA jackets. All the president needs to do is declare a national emergency, and then FEMA becomes your GOD. It's as simple as that. What's wrong with that? Well, you can kiss the law of the land good-bye, the constitution of these united states, and the bill of rights; they will be gone as long as the president declares there is a national emergency. The constitution is OFFICIALLY suspended indefinitely until further notice. Each state has it's own version of FEMA, all of which include the following laws which take effect immediately upon the declaration of an emergency: The CDC declares the emergency whenever they want to, and the president enacts FEMA.

:THE BOTTOM LINE WILL BECOME:

When federal and state public health officials convince your governor to declare a "public health emergency," they will have the authority to use the state militia to:

➤ Take control of all roads leading into and out of your cities and state.

➤ Seize your house, car, telephones, computers, food, fuel, clothing, firearms, and alcoholic beverages for their own use, and not be held liable if these actions result in the destruction of your personal property.

➤ Arrest and imprison you or any member of your family, including your CHILDREN for any reason they see fit, and forcibly examine, vaccinate and medicate you and your children without your consent, and not be held liable if these actions result in your death, or your child's death or injury as a result of such actions.

My good friends please hear me fully! These FEMA regulations have been around for over 25 years just waiting for an emergency.

And now the CDC is pushing hard daily to get smallpox vaccination laws, as well as many others into effect, administered by FEMA. All they need do after that is declare an emergency, and we all know how easy it will be for the CDC to declare an emergency whenever they desire. A few plants of smallpox here or there is all it will take, then **BOOM**

Welcome to Amerika, the Fascist Nation

There will be no rhyme or reason; no questions to be asked. You will be monitored like a pet dog with a computerized vaccination card; perhaps even a mandatory subcutaneous chip implant. Just like your dog or cat, if you haven't had all your shots, you will be denied travel, hotel stays, and most assuredly imprisoned until you comply. Forget the mile high piles of research that prove vaccines are dangerous; forget any scientific studies about the effectiveness of a smallpox vaccine, or for that matter any vaccine. Medical historians have shown that the smallpox epidemic of the early 20th century was a sham. Statistics were altered, and misdiagnosis ran rampant all to show a favorable result for smallpox vaccines. People were dying from the ill effects of many unsanitary conditions of that time, and it was all called "smallpox." History shows that the smallpox vaccine campaigns of the early 20th century were met with very poor compliance; the chance of dying from smallpox was far greater if you received the vaccine than if you did nothing at all. What has been suppressed by the pharmaceutical cartel is that smallpox was nearly eradicated by the time the vaccine was pushed on the public.

Doesn't common sense tell us that if vaccines really do work, than those who choose to receive vaccines will not be at any risk from those who choose not to be vaccinated? Why does the CDC need to install a state militia governed by a totalitarian FEMA to force people to be vaccinated? Especially when you consider that most people don't believe what I am saying here, think I am totally nuts, and will fight to be one of the first on line to receive their vaccine!

The answer is simple. Because the CDC is well aware that their vaccines are total shams and toxic; blunders that actually create more disease and suffering than they prevent. Here is the God's honest solid point of the entire matter;

You simply can't have a lot of totally healthy UNVACCINATED people walking around, telling others they never received their shots, when many people who have received the vaccines get sick and die. This is very bad for business.

By forcing EVERYONE to be vaccinated, they can assuredly place credit to their vaccine for everyone who survives and say "too bad" for all those who die, that dreaded disease got'em despite all our best minds and efforts. Let us pray.

Believe me folks;

They fully realize unvaccinated people will be far healthier than anyone who receives the vaccine, and they will never study this fact. To have healthy unvaccinated people walking and talking about is a solid statement of conviction to their fraud. They need to vaccinate everyone for one purpose only; to destroy the evidence that vaccines are killing and maiming people.

Of course pharmaceutical companies do not want to study unvaccinated populations. To do this would open them up to tremendous scrutiny and liability. Can you just imagine what this would do to them?! They would cease to exist if everyone knew the truth, and that is precisely why they are expending a ton of energy RIGHT NOW to get these laws passed in every state.

God rest the souls of 9-11. The media and government spin the tragedy to the American public as something totally different from what it really is; from what it has always been, and the real reason it all happened in the first place;

A mega-tool for the Illuminati elite to CASH in. A grand
opportunity to crush all competition in commerce, especially in
the middle east and related specifically to oil, the dollar over the
euro, and other valuable natural resources; to promote a ONE
WORLD agenda, a ONE WORLD banking system with no
outside competition, and a ONE WORLD police state; to place
big corporations, governments and their leaders in a greater
position to run your life, by stealing away the most basic of
freedoms you were granted as a birthright by being born in
America. If you don't have the freedom to decide what you are to
do with your own body, it is difficult to decipher what freedoms
you actually do have.

Has anyone read even a small portion of the new "**Patriot Bills
I & II?**" An elementary school student can see that these bills have
absolutely NOTHING to do with protecting you from terrorists.
The provisions of these bills give full police power to the Attorney
General, to incarcerate YOU indefinitely if he deems you are a
terrorist by any means! Even if a state judge releases you from jail,
the Attorney General can rescind that release and keep you in the
slammer as long as he wants! The bill takes away all DUE PROCESS
of law for ANYONE that is even suspect of being associated with
terrorism. You are totally guilty if the Attorney General says you
are, and you must prove your innocence. You can be arrested for
terrorism for merely participating in an anti-war demonstration
(of which you will be seeing many in the coming months, mark
my word). I can be arrested for terrorism by simply writing this
book! I can be arrested for terrorism by simply guiding you to
think for yourself, and fight back against being forcefully vaccinated.
The Patriot Bill is a total sham, and is better labeled the *Fascist
Bill.* Read it for yourself and find out. It is available on the internet
at a few sites.

What to do? If you've actually read this far, I commend you.
80% of the American population will lay quietly to the propaganda
and gleefully waltz to the FEMA vaccination stations. Another
10% will bitch and moan about it, and succumb out of fear. The

remaining 10%, like myself, will fight with everything they have to protect their God given common law right to do as they please with their bodies, and to protect their children as they see fit from dangerous chemicals being injected directly into the bloodstream. So since you are still reading, here are some things I can suggest;

➤ Immediately if not sooner, call the National Vaccine Information Center (NVIC), @ 1-800-909-SHOT, or visit them on line @ *www.909shot.com*. Call them and join today. They need money to keep people and a few honest lawmakers informed.

➤ Research as many vaccine reality and truth sites as you are able. Here are some presently available:

http://www.vaccinationnews.com
http://www.whale.to/vaccines.html
http://www.nccn.net/~wwithin/vaccine.htm
http://www.909shot.com
http://www.thinktwice.com
http://www.redflagsweekly.com
http://home.san.rr.com/via/
http://www.vaccine-info.com

➤ Call or write your federal and state legislators! Tell them you are outraged by the thought of such laws.

➤ Write the same outrage to the Attorney General, and whatever Health Secretary Bozo is presently masquerading as a public servant as well as the President and first lady. Tell them you insist on biological freedom.

Talk to as many people as you can about this issue and it's ramifications. Keep communicating and keep active in the fight for health care and biological freedom.

Chapter Six
Historical Chicanery

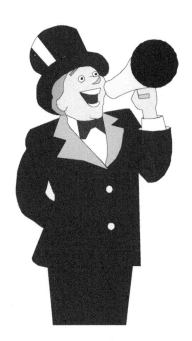

All of recorded history regarding disease has been altered to point the finger at micro-organisms as the cause. However, regardless of widespread belief in the germ theory 50 years ago, it was nonetheless common knowledge that good hygiene and a balanced diet was the main contributor to disease prevention. Especially since the 1970's, the medical cartel has bombarded Americans with its' propaganda, to the extent where text books are changed to only reveal the medical party line, and the entire focus is taken off of prevention. *Historically, one will discover that better hygiene, improved dietary habits and natural cycles have been the true reasons for the reversed cycles of certain major diseases.* But through its' immense influence in government and propaganda, the medical cartel has grabbed all the credit for this reduction in disease. Imagine what it would be like if cigarette manufacturers were allowed to continue their advertising on television and radio, like they did in the old days of broadcasting. Today, at the beginning of the twenty first century, we may well believe that cigarettes actually provide vital nutrition absorbed through the lungs! We could have been led to believe that cigarette smoking should be taken up as early as possible to develop strong, healthy lungs. Sound ridiculous? This very principle is exactly what the medical cartel has been allowed to bombard us with over the past 50 years. The net result is that we are a far weaker, less vital and more diseased people than we were 50 years before this massive and obtrusive medical influence.

Next time your pediatrician boasts the wonders of medical vaccination programs that have eradicated once major and devastating diseases, pull her head up from bowing to the floor by her photo of Jonas Salk, and let her know you have some knowledge to share. The AMA, like a greedy politician, makes a business of taking credit for things they didn't do. Here's the truth people: *All of the major diseases that the Medical cartel claims to have eradicated were on the decline already by natural forces, improved self health care (like better nutrition), and improved education on sanitation and hygiene.* Nearly *90%* of the total decline in death rate in children between 1860 and 1965 due to whooping cough, scarlet fever, diphtheria, and measles occurred before the onset of antibiotics, and wide spread immunization programs.

With regards to all these old statistics used by the pharmaceutical companies in the 1950's and 1960's to "prove" vaccines wiped out the disease they were given for, the reader needs to understand as fundamental knowledge that all these early statistics from 1880 to 1965 showed a huge decline in disease incidence *NOT* due the administration of any vaccine, but due to advancements at this time in sanitation and public hygiene; i.e., less crowding of living spaces, better nutritional education, cleaner running water, plumbing for bath, shower and human waste. A generalized increase in the quality of living conditions occurred at this time in the history of western civilization, and these early, very dirty pharmaceutical companies jumped in to take credit for the health these things produced, stating it was due to their products that humanity was now saved from the scourge of these diseases. Every time the medical cartel quotes an example of how great vaccination programs are, they will do so using a statistic from 1910 to 1930, stating that thousands of children were dying of the said diseases at this time. Whereas this is true, looking at any graph from 1880 to 1970 will show that 1910/1930 disease rates were already on a steep decline from the earlier years as public hygiene and the sanitation industry grew.

Vaccination programs for the mass public were not introduced until the mid 1950's in all cases you research; not until the tail end of the graph when the disease was decreased by over 90% from the beginning of the graph period (usually beginning at 1880 to 1900).

When considering the psychological profile of the parents and grandparents from that time period between 1950 and 1970; the one's whose children (like me) received the prototypical dosages of mass vaccination, you can understand how easily they were fooled. Mostly all of them were traumatized from either the direct experience, memory or story of some family member who was maimed, paralyzed or killed from one of the dreaded diseases. Now here come these pharmaceutical representatives, fully understanding this psychological climate and taking full advantage of it's effects on local and federal government officials. Far less people had any of these diseases, but fear of them still reined free and true. Now here come the saviors! Those altruistic and hard working medical scientists, who will save society and quell your fears about these terrible things happening to you or your children. These early pharmaceutical representatives were nothing more than the progeny of snake oil salesman from the turn of the 20th century. You can just picture them there in the early days, standing on their soap boxes in the middle of the road; *"Just one shot my good friends will give you all the protection and peace of mind you need! You don't need to do anything else! We'll take care of you and your family from this point forward!"* Well, we all know how that "protection" truly worked out now, don't we. More disease instead of less, as those very diseases were already fully declined. More heartache and loss with the birth of a generation of neurologically and brain damaged children, directly caused by their "cures."

The standard M.O. for disguising their fraud throughout these early years of mass vaccination horror, a practice which occurs still to this day in the 21st century, was to train doctors and other medical cartel representatives *not to diagnose the said disease any more after the vaccination programs were administered, even if the exact same symptoms showed up in medical offices after the shots were administered. If it looked like polio after the polio shot was given, it just couldn't be polio anymore. It had to be something that a vaccine was not given for like spinal meningitis. If it looked like measles, it just couldn't be anymore. It had to be an allergic rash of some form or another. This practice alone of manually altering statistics and reporting is responsible for much of the public confusion centered around mass vaccination programs today, and the sole reason they are still promoted as gospel.*

Public officials always declare doom and gloom would be the result if vaccination programs were to stop. But experience tells us something different. Typically when pertussis vaccination is decreased in different parts of the world, as was done in 1981 by Sweden and the U.K., pertussis death rates actually dropped dramatically in both countries, England reporting the lowest death rates in recorded history. More whooping cough was diagnosed in these areas during this period however, and this is another fine example of how a promoted psychological climate from the medical cartel alters reality, and creates a false sense of trouble favorable for their products. When it was introduced that pertussis vaccination programs would be decreased or eliminated as a test, medical and pharmaceutical cartel representatives spread panic by insisting doctors look for a probable whooping cough (same as pertussis) outbreak. Due to this panic, now every case of bronchitis and flu that enters into the doctors office suddenly becomes whooping cough. Due to the subjective nature of data recording in these instances, increases in any specific disease are virtually meaningless since you can't be certain which problem you are actually talking about. In most cases throughout the world, doctors will refuse to diagnose a disease in which a person has been vaccinated for. This political bias alone is enough to alter statistics persistently showing a false yet favorable result for vaccines.

"When vaccination rates drop, every time the child clears his throat the pediatrician will diagnose whooping cough."
Robert Mendelsohn, MD

How does anyone know how many children and adults are truly getting "sick?" Truth of the matter is, **there is no real and honest way of confirming disease reporting in today's world dominated by the medical cartel.** In every case of disease reporting there can be a huge variation between cases subjectively diagnosed and those objectively confirmed. Statistics for disease are compiled for government by medical professionals that have a vested financial interest in vaccination programs, either directly administered by their medical offices or by indirectly promoting a product, like a vaccine, in which they own stock. Laboratory confirmations are not required by the FDA or any other office of government to confirm disease rates; medical doctors can virtually diagnose whatever they want without check, and this becomes part of "official" statistics!

In February 2002 a study was done in England to do just this, confirm by laboratory testing what medical doctors were diagnosing as measles. The result? The diagnoses were found to be 99% inaccurate by laboratory confirmation. What does all this mean? Clearly, we have the Fox guarding the hen house. Those who have a vested financial interest in vaccination programs are given carte blanche authority to declare a need for prevention of diseases that don't even exist.

It is a well known fact that polio was decreasing very well on it's own as well before the mandated vaccination programs. In Europe where the vaccine was hardly used, this was also the case. In America polio increased dramatically in the 1950's after the vaccination program for polio was administered. Shortly afterwards once again, if people began showing up with polio symptoms after they had their shot, they were diagnosed with spinal meningitis, even with paralysis! If they did not have their shot they were diagnosed with polio. How convenient.

The CDC publishes a chart each year on the state of "infectious" disease in the United States. They only chart these diseases since 1955 however. When I called them, they told me they had no records prior to 1955. Isn't that interesting!? Why do you suppose this is so? The CDC does not want you to see that if you track disease back to the early 1900's, long before antibiotics, medications and vaccines were so powerfully on the scene, all of the above mentioned diseases were already 90% diminished from their peak levels. This is a crime of fraud that should be punishable by our most basic laws.

By it's own admission, the government realizes that despite the enormous level of reporting which lead to the formation of VAERS, there is still a lot that goes unreported or re-diagnosed (as apposed to mis-diagnosed, which is not intentional). Many children show up with neurological damage and other related problems following vaccines, but the MD convinces the parent that vaccines had nothing to do with the problem. The FDA has stated that; *"doctors under-report adverse vaccine reactions by 90%."*

In 1973, *Scientific America* published a research article in one of their popular magazines, showing that between 1900 and 1950 declining death rates were obvious in TB and typhoid. During this time there was no vaccine for TB. It declined naturally like all other infectious diseases had during this time.

The pertussis vaccine has been reported to be about 50% effective. But what does this mean? It means that about 50% of *vaccinated people* still get the disease. Why do you suppose this is a fact? In 1978, 8,092 cases of whooping cough were reported in the British Medical Journal, and discussed at the International Symposium on pertussis in Bethesda Maryland. Of these 8,092, 36% were vaccinated, 30% were unvaccinated and 34% were not recorded with a doctor. It is a fact of medical history that malnutrition, poor natal and obstetric care, and the poor, unsanitary living conditions of the late 19th and early 20th centuries improved rapidly after 1948 world wide. The health of children thus world wide reflected these improved conditions. Between the years of 1850 and 1950, records of morbidity and mortality became more available in the United Kingdom, and they found that the child population had increased enormously. Also during this time, incidence of death from whooping cough decreased from over 1,000 to less than 10 cases per million. The same can be said for measles, diphtheria, scarlet fever and TB. It is clearly seen from these and other reliable statistics that 90% of the decline of these infectious diseases occurred before the advent of vaccination programs, prior to 1950. Based on statistics and research compiled by independent researchers in the United Kingdom, it was found that *over 45% of whooping cough cases after the onset of vaccinations occurred in fully vaccinated children.*

Party Line #5:   The great polio epidemic of the late 1940's and
early 1950's was finally eradicated by our
national hero, Jonas Salk, who's Salk vaccine for
polio saved us all. Due to his vaccine, polio is
virtually non-existent in today's world.

Polio is probably the disease which is used most to describe
the efficacy of a vaccine program to wipe out an epidemic, but
nothing can be further from the truth. Jonas Salk, the developer of
the polio vaccine is hailed as a national hero. Interestingly enough,
*Jonas Salk made a public statement in 1976 that two thirds of the
cases of polio that occurred between 1966 and 1976 were caused
by his vaccine.* Isn't that interesting. There are many inconsistencies
regarding data surrounding this disease, polio. According to
nationwide statistics, polio decreased from 18,000 cases in 1954,
to fewer than 20 cases in 1973-78. This sounds like something
good happened to wipe out this awful disease. But if you read
between the lines, you find something very different happened. At
a congressional hearing on the subject in 1978, Dr. Bernard
Greenberg reported that not only did the incidence of polio *increase*
substantially after the introduction of mass and frequently
compulsory vaccination programs, but statistics were manipulated,
and false statements were made by the National Public Health
Service to give the opposite impression. Details on this can be
obtained by reading the congressional hearings on HR 10541.

In 1957, the North Carolina Health Department made
glowing claims for the efficacy of the Salk vaccine, showing that
polio steadily decreased there from 1953 to 1957 after public
vaccination. However, these figures were challenged by Dr. Fred
Clenner of North Carolina, who pointed out that it wasn't until
1955 that a single person in his state even received the polio Vaccine.
Even then, the number of injections were administered on a very
limited basis, because of the number of polio cases which actually

resulted from the vaccine! It wasn't until 1956 that polio vaccinations became widespread in North Carolina. This 61% drop in polio therefore, was credited to the Salk vaccine when it wasn't even in the state yet! Nevertheless, by 1957, when massive vaccination programs were instituted, polio was again on the increase. If one checks the details of most states that still have their data on record, this kind of chicanery is widespread.

There are many ways, besides the above, in which polio statistics were manipulated to give the impression of the effectiveness of the Salk vaccine. Before the onset of the polio vaccine program, the diagnostic parameter classifying an epidemic was 20 cases of polio per 100,000 population. Immediately after the polio vaccine program began however, this parameter was conveniently switched to 35 cases of polio per 100,000. Nearly a 75% increase in the number of cases necessary to classify a polio epidemic! This in and of itself would throw out the chance of any further polio "epidemics." Nothing changed except for the criteria the government and medical professionals now used to name the disease. The disease polio was also redefined medically after the onset of the vaccine. Before the vaccine, to be diagnosed as having paralytic poliomyelitis, one had to have paralytic symptoms for 24 hours. After the vaccine, this was changed to 60 days! That's quite a jump, wouldn't you say?! By changing the diagnostic parameter in this way, a doctor could almost say good-bye to what he used to know as polio. People still came in with polio like symptoms, but now the doctor couldn't call it polio any more. He had to find another name for it, like a bad flu or more likely, *spinal meningitis.* This simple change in definition meant that in 1955, we started reporting a new disease, which usually was paralytic poliomyelitis with a longer lasting paralysis, and some other new name. After the introduction of the Salk vaccine, aseptic spinal meningitis was now distinctly different from polio. Playing the angle on this dirty game from both ends, before the vaccine, in 1954, many cases that were actually aseptic spinal meningitis were diagnosed as polio. Isn't that convenient! The symptomatology of these two supposedly different diseases are essentially identical. Wherever records are kept in every state health department, you will discover that during the onset of the polio vaccine as incidence of polio decreased, spinal meningitis increased proportionately. Polio and spinal meningitis are the same disease, separated and brought together for the convenience of the researcher.

When challenged on this point, the United States Department of Health, Education and Welfare responded;

"The reason aseptic meningitis was reported separately [from Polio] is that most cases of aseptic meningitis observed by clinicians up to the early 1950's were considered non-paralytic poliomyelitis, or meningitis of an obscure etiology . . . ."

This is total nonsense and double talk. How do you think they came to this conclusion, and conclusions like this regarding polio? By using the same stupidity they always use when defining disease rates. They assume it can't be polio because they vaccinated against it already, and they assume the vaccine is totally effective without fail or question. Similar nonsense happens with most so called "communicable" disease reporting data. In this case, it was ridiculously assumed that polio **HAD TO DECLINE** from the vaccine program, so all those new cases of polio that were found after the vaccine program couldn't possibly be polio. This is like assuming a person takes on a totally new physical identity after a baptism. It's all up to the personal beliefs, motivated for whatever reasons, of the believer.

The CDC responded on this subject as follows;

"When the laboratory techniques allowed for culturing the viruses related to aseptic meningitis in the mid 1950's, it became clear that the vast majority of aseptic meningitis was caused by enteroviruses other than polio. Therefore in the late 1950's it was decided that aseptic meningitis, presumably due to other enteroviruses other than polio, be reported separately from poliomyelitis."

That's it folks! It just became clear! They saw the light, and the religion of medicine moved on further with their doctrine of vaccination. You know how they saw the light? Because they vaccinated against polio, and the vaccinations could do no harm, and just had to work. They assume this today, despite overwhelming evidence to the contrary.

Despite all this nonsense, polio increases were reported before and after the vaccination programs in Tennessee, Ohio, Connecticut and North Carolina. You can check this for yourself. In Tennessee, 119 cases were reported before the vaccine program, and 386 cases were reported after. In Ohio, there were 17 cases before, and 52 cases after. In Connecticut there were 45 cases before, and 123 after. In North Carolina there were 78 before, and 313 cases after. But trust them folks. They'll always tell you to get down on your knees and believe in the vaccine, because it "works." Who exactly does it work for?

In school, you never learned of the *other two polio epidemics* seen by the United States. You were told there was only one just prior to the vaccine in which we were all saved by Jonas Salk. The truth is, that there was one in the teens and one in the thirties, and for some reason both of them just went away naturally. The reason for this is that there were no vaccines back then keeping the disease going longer than it had to. Polio disappeared in Europe in the forties and fifties all on its' own, without vaccines. It also virtually disappeared in the United States before the vaccine program, which actually had the opposite effect of its' intent.

One interesting fact regarding polio, is that is soared astronomically around 1948. Do you know what this correlates with? This was the time of compulsory vaccine programs for diphtheria, which created polio in once again epidemic proportions. After this, it naturally declined once again as people got healthier, and free from these vaccines. Then came the said polio vaccine programs, which once again made the incidence of polio shoot through the roof. Then it naturally declined once again, but this time the medical cartel took credit for it, and began a campaign of advertising propaganda second to none. Due to this, you will find very few people in the United States who believe anything other than the medical party line on the history of polio.

Dr. Alec Burton sums this all up nicely with his quote from the Natural Hygiene Society's Milwaukee meeting in 1978;

"It is a fact that statistics were compiled which show that the polio vaccine in use at the time had no influence what so ever on the polio epidemic at large. Data from New South Wales and Australia shows that polio occurs in cycles anyway. When it has been "conquered" by vaccines, and a disease with identical symptoms continues to appear, doctors look for a new virus because they assume the old one has been wiped out."

Party Line #6:	Small Pox was wiped out by mass vaccination campaigns after tedious years of dedicated research.

"It is pathetic and ludicrous to say we ever vanquished smallpox with vaccines, when only 10% of the population was ever vaccinated."
—*Glen Dettman, MD*

Small pox was actually created by mass vaccination campaigns. An 1895 entry in the *Encyclopedia Britannica*, written by Dr. Charles Craten, actually tore the small pox vaccination program to pieces from his own research. He also noted a strange "coincidence" between small pox vaccinations, and occurrences of syphilis in children whose parents did not have syphilis. These findings created so much outrage at the time, that they were never printed again.

Sir Alfred Russel Wallace, a prominent researcher of his time, wrote in chapter 18 of his 1899 book, *"The Wonderful Century;"*

"Vaccinations are a delusion, and its' penile enforcement is a crime."

This chapter contains pages upon pages of data he obtained from researching all the available morbidity and mortality records of his time. The conclusion was that the small pox vaccination was a complete fraud, which caused more small pox than it cured.

Even the esteemed author George Bernard Shaw wrote;

"During the last considerable epidemic of small pox during the turn of the century, I was a member of the health committee of Londonboro council, and I learned how the credit of vaccination is kept up statistically by diagnosing all the vaccinated cases of small pox as "pustular exema," amongst other things. Anything but small pox."

Certainly the Small Pox vaccine is a prime example of one routine shot, which was eventually discontinued when the morbidity, or occurrence of the disease from the vaccine itself far exceeded its' benefits. Australia and New Zealand were practically unvaccinated at the time, and were more free from small pox than any other country. The most thoroughly vaccinated countries were Italy, the Philippines, Mexico and the former British India. All of these nations to the contrary, were scourged with small pox. After the U.S. vaccine program hit the Philippines, they actually experienced the largest epidemic of small pox to ever hit their country. 162,000 cases and 71,000 deaths were reported in vaccinated people. Now you know why they love us in the Philippines.

Japan began compulsory small pox vaccinations in 1872, and continued it for about 100 years with disastrous results. By 1892, their records showed 165,000 cases with over 29,000 deaths in vaccinated people. In Australia, where there were no compulsory small pox vaccinations, there were only 3 deaths in 15 years! You do the math.

Party Line #7:   The syphilis outbreaks of the 1940's, 50's and 60's were experienced most severely by service men in the Navy. This was a result of the men being on ship for extended periods of time, and philandering quite a bit when they finally got to shore. Much of this philandering was done with prostitutes who either had syphilis or were syphilitic carriers.

Although this party line is not entirely incorrect, one must remember that the more poignant correlating factor with these military personnel, is that enlisted men and women are required to receive a myriad of vaccines; much more than the average civilian. These vaccines are responsible for hundreds of health problems experienced by our service personnel over their lifetime. The government is quick to point the blame elsewhere, as usual.

Party Line #8:   Measles outbreaks were finally brought under control by vaccine programs. From 1958 to 1966, the decline of measles was approximately 800,000 childhood cases to 200,000.

Well, it sounds good, but what they don't tell us is that measles already had a decline of about 90% from 1948 to 1958. But the CDC will still insist that vaccines have wiped out measles, and preach this to all local health departments. Their charts and data show that the measles vaccine was licensed in 1963, and from this point the incidence of the disease shot way down. However, what they again don't tell us, is that *the measles vaccine did not receive widespread use until 1967.* From the party line above you can see how much the disease had already declined before this use. The first batch of measles vaccine that was used in 1963, upon licensing, was quickly eliminated due to horrific side effects. The medical cartel took total credit for the decline of measles, even though it had already declined well before widespread use of their failed vaccines.

If you investigate measles back to 1900, you will find that the disease had already begun to decline way back then. It only began to spike up again when vaccine programs for other diseases became more prevalent in the 1950's. The CDC also claims that during the 1991 measles "epidemic," most children who came down with the disease were unvaccinated. *Notice that the CDC will never claim a category of children who did not come down with any disease while being unvaccinated.* The term "MOST" is a misleading generality the CDC uses often in its' reporting. To them, "MOST" could mean 51%. This also means that they are claiming, quite noncommittally, that a certain portion of the vaccinated population actually gets the disease they have been vaccinated against. They place no energy in the scientific study of why certain unvaccinated children do not get sick. Ever wonder why?

Sadly enough, most of the incidence of contagious disease "outbreaks" that you hear about are constructed, whether or not intentionally . . . . I dare not say. There is actually an epidemic intelligence service (EIS) of the CDC. A group of employees who are hired to go here and there, looking for clusters of symptoms they can run back to the CDC with and call an epidemic. Seek and Ye shall find, but why don't these same people receive training in how to locate the vast portion of the population which stays healthy around their clusters of "epidemics?"

During the Gulf war, I heard stories from enlisted people of friends who actually dropped dead, or went into anaphylactic shock, after receiving massive levels of vaccines all at once. Many soldiers came back from the Persian Gulf quite ill. It wasn't all from chemical poisoning, as the public has been mislead to believe. It turns out, that during the Gulf war soldiers were given an experimental anthrax vaccine for fear of biological warfare. Although data on this subject has been suppressed by the military and government, I will bet it all on vaccines being the primary cause of sickness amongst these soldiers. These ill soldiers have been the subject of many a television news special, and the VA will claim everything but vaccines as the culprit behind their woes. One of my favorites was PTSD, or Post Traumatic Stress Disorder (a psychological disorder formally known as "shell shock" during W.W.II). This is exactly what they told the Vietnam vets when they came back from the war with dioxin poisoning. Another good one was that these ill Gulf War military personnel were showering in water that had become contaminated with petroleum, and hence they developed petroleum poisoning. The tumors and arthritis these enlisted men and women obtained from the vaccines could not possibly have been caused by petroleum poisoning. This data, easily correlating vaccines to disease in the military is simply suppressed from the public. Due to this, the only way proper research can be done is to adequately study these ill military personnel, applying simple and honest scientific facts.

When will it ever be done? Not until enough of us know the truth and speak out about it loud enough. Until that time, this trend of historical chicanery will continue.

Chapter Seven
Immunity or Lunacy?

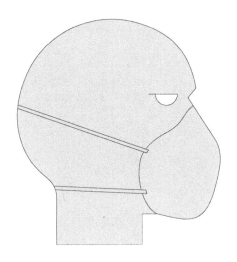

We are taught in school an antiquated version of so called, "immunity" which is increasingly loosing credibility in many scientific arenas around the globe. The entire notion that antibody titers (counts that occur through blood tests) can solidify a diagnosis for some disease has no basis in rational science. Nor does the notion that the presence of antibodies will prevent any given disease. Antibodies go up in the blood for one reason alone, and that is *toxemia*. The theory that one has to have a disease first to be *immune* from that disease ever happening again, all to the credit of antibody production, is about as smart as believing that you have to get burned first in order to prevent future burning.

To begin, we must take a rational look at what exactly immunity is. Immunity is a defense system the body uses to *eliminate toxic matter* that has built up over a period of time. The immune system is wonderfully complex, and kicks into place when more simple lines of body defense have not been able to eliminate toxic matter effectively, and now the toxicity has reached the circulatory system and organs. There are varying forms of white blood cells which are the immune system's primary line of defense in regards to this elimination. Antibodies then, are specially synthesized body proteins which aid the white blood cells when toxicity reaches more extreme levels. I have sifted through a ton of data, and thus challenge anyone to present a single piece of evidence which proves antibodies are produced to defend against so called "germs."

We've all seen microscopic photos of the valiant white blood cells undergoing phagocytosis (surrounding and engulfing) of said germs, but this is not what is happening in these photos. The white blood cells are simply removing dead organic matter, or garbage, from the body that is no longer useful. These so called germs are not attacking the body to make it sick in benefit solely for itself. In fact, that is the definition of a *parasite*, and parasitic infestations and infections are possible. But microbes like bacteria have a useful function for the body, and when they die off, they are consumed by white blood cells simply as a clean up process.

In reality, there **is no immunity from germs**, because germs are not the culprit opportunists they are made out to be, causing everyone they come into contact with to get sick. You've been told that vaccines stimulate antibody production, and these antibodies will protect you when and if the real disease comes along. However, there are children born with the disorder, *agammaglobulinemia*, which simply means they cannot produce gamma globulin's, the chief proteins constituting antibodies. Therefore, they cannot make any antibodies. These are the famous "bubble kids," since many of them live within ridiculous (loved that *Bubble Boy* Seinfeld Episode!) artificial latex walls to limit exposure from the dirty world of germs outside. The children with this disorder who do not live in bubbles however (and there have been many), *are still able to recover from measles and other diseases as spontaneously as normal children.* Why is this? Why has it not been adequately researched? The answer is simple. You don't need antibodies to recover from any disease, and the medical cartel knows it. Antibody tests, detection and stimulation products however are the central hub of their fraudulent wheel. To remove this hub is to collapse the entire scam pushed upon the world for decades.

Antibodies have never been a scientifically proven relief of impending and harmful disease. Their presence does not guarantee you will be safe from any particular disease, in fact. There is a good amount of research still available to prove this point. In the *British Medical Research Council Report #272* from May of 1950, there is an outline of a study on diphtheria done in the north of England. This study tested the correlation between antibody counts in people who were treating diphtheria patients, and the patients themselves. The study found that there was no correlation what so ever between antibody count in the individual, and their ability to develop diphtheria antigens (which simply means getting diphtheria). In other words, there were people with diphtheria with very low antibody counts, and some with very high. Other people who were attending these ill ones had extremely low antibody counts. Due to this lack of correlation between antibody and disease, the study was terminated and called a failure.

Think about this well for a moment. If a research company does not come up with the expected results, for example, to prove a correlation between antibodies and disease, how long do you suppose they will stay in business? Do you think the pharmaceutical companies will pay them for any further research projects? Or in the case of University research, how long will the grant money keep flowing if the expected lab results are not forthcoming? The obvious answer is, not very long. *Dr. Peter Duesberg*, a prestigious University professor and viral researcher for decades, has been attempting to tell people the truth about AIDS for 10 years. He went on national television and told the interviewer, that he would drink up an HIV viral infested cup of coffee right in front of him if asked to, without any fear of becoming ill, because his research had unequivocally found no correlation what so ever between the culprit HIV virus, and the disease AIDS. He was totally ostracized from the research community for it, although many colleagues went on record to say Duesberg was quite correct. They just didn't want to be the ones to say it, and loose *their* research grants. In medicine, the result of research all too often comes down to the mighty power of the buck. Who's paying for it?

Why do they want a certain level of results? These are the first questions that should always be asked regarding medical and pharmaceutical research. "Medical research" thus, can become nothing more than an elaborate form of propaganda. If you want the truth, you can find it. But you need to have the drive to look beneath the lies, and my experience has been that very few people are willing to make this effort.

In spite of the party line that antibodies are indicative of a protective reaction to disease, a very marked immunity exists without their presence. It has been proven time and time again that the mere presence of antibodies cannot confirm a diagnosis of disease, nor insure protection from it. Bacteriologists and other researchers have known this fact for a long time. Then again, if you've vested a tremendous amount of time and money in medical school, or if you require grant money for your research business, one can very easily from a stance of mindless practicality follow the germ theory party line. This is done with a fairly clean conscience, since there is plenty of material to support the theory that germs are the causative factors in disease. As time goes on however, doctors of medicine are requiring larger and larger blinders to keep themselves from the truth. Antibodies should totally be stripped of their immense importance, since they are at best, a secondary line of body defense.

Party Line #10: AIDS was discovered in 1982. It is a terrible disease, highly infectious through sexual contact, and caused by infection of the HIV virus, which destroys a persons' white blood cell line of defense. Thus, a persons' immune system is severely compromised, leaving one virtually defenseless against the world's most common pathogens, where a simple cold can become a life threatening disease. Without treatment, death is immanent.

To begin to tell you the truth about AIDS, a major piece of epidemic propaganda pushed on the American public, and the world by the CDC, let's first state that AIDS is simply a redefinition of an old disease called *leukocytopenia*. If you research old versions of the Merck manual, as well as older diagnostic texts, you will find that leukocytopenia, meaning simply decreased white blood cells, was purposely graduated to *"Acquired Immune Deficiency Syndrome"* at a press conference held by the CDC in 1982. Leukocytopenia has identical symptoms to AIDS, and was not considered a sexually transmitted disease, but a disease of toxicity caused from drugs and environmental toxins. The CDC claimed in 1982, without any confirmatory research, that HIV was the cause of this sexually transmitted disease now called AIDS, which at present was occurring primarily in homosexual men. They also made reference to Haitians and Africans who most likely brought the HIV virus to America. For years, the public bought this hook, line and sinker. This was to be the CDC's propaganda masterpiece, but fortunately for us, it backfired due to the outspoken research of many a good and honest University researcher, such as *Peter Duesberg* who we have already mentioned. The results of their research, showing that AIDS could not possibly be caused by HIV, was the subject of many a prime time television show in the early 1990's. AIDS has certainly lost its' death sentence since then, but not from any form of medical treatment. It happened from a public who educated themselves and began to search for the truth on their own. People were coming down with the diagnosis all over the globe, from the erroneous HIV antibody test which could show a Catholic Nun to have the HIV virus. This test is still in effect today, ruining peoples' lives with the stigma of a false disease.

Many companies require their employees to have regular AIDS tests, and whether or not you come up with the diagnosis has much to do with the luck of the draw, but quite more to do with how clean your blood is. People who are in a high state of detoxification, with or without symptoms, usually wind up testing positive for the so called *"AIDS antibodies."* This state of detoxification could have nothing to do with how "clean" you live your life in the conventional sense, i.e., you don't drink and you don't use recreational drugs. Most people have high levels of blood toxicity primarily due to faulty dietary habits, as well as prescribed and over the counter types of medications. The all too common scenario with AIDS is that people test positive for the antibody when they feel fine, they panic and run to their doctor, and he places them on AZT and / or another terrible anti viral drug. The person then undoubtedly begins to have symptoms which are attributed to the progression of AIDS, when in actuality they are created from the poisonous medications they now have in their blood stream.

I have also read stories which attempted to prove that the *actual* AIDS virus was genetically engineered and administered upon the gay population as an experiment, which was to blame the gays for beginning a world wide, AIDS epidemic. Could this be true? Well, there is certainly no hard proof of this claim, and if it is true they evidently failed miserably at it (this time anyway). The way governments run these days, and considering the out of control power available to the medical cartel, I wouldn't doubt it. But the proof is always difficult to come by since tracks in this kind of conspiracy are generally well covered. The story goes that during the height of the cold war, a Polish nationalist doctor and viral researcher was allowed mysteriously with his wife and children to attend a medical conference in Italy. What is obviously strange about this to anyone who lived through that time in history, is that all members of a family were never allowed to leave a communist block nation at the same time for fear of defection. Why come back if you could defect all of your family to the West for freedom? This is exactly what happened next. He and his entire family defected, and within a few years he wound up head researcher at the NY Blood Center. Sounds very curious, but nonetheless . . . . He supposedly sponsored a very experimental hepatitis B vaccine program in New York City, Chicago and San Francisco. All their major papers then ran ads for gay men to try the new vaccine in 1971 and 1972. About 10 years later is when the major outbreaks of AIDS began in those very cities.

I am by no means asserting here that antibody tests are "rigged," so to say, in order to provide an ample business population for medical professionals. Although I would not doubt this to be true in some of the cases, I mostly acknowledge that medical professionals really believe their antibody tests confirm disease. This is due to a general lack of education on the part of medical professionals, in the comprehension of any other way of thinking besides what has been taught in medical school. The truth is, these antibody tests are most likely testing for a generalized level of blood toxicity due to poor dietary habits, prescribed and over the counter medications. Antibodies do have a purpose in the body, and that is a secondary line of defense to white blood cells in the systematic clean up of body garbage. This is primarily the clean up of large protein molecules that have made their way into the blood and intercellular fluids. These large protein molecules, and the antibodies created to eliminate them, are what create the "positive" antibody test result for any given disease. From this information, medical professionals usually misunderstand the tests' true meaning, and connect the dots of their limited education to form some party line diagnosis.

AIDS is a classic example of flawed CDC propaganda. There are so many inconsistencies surrounding AIDS, its diagnosis and treatment, that I would doubt a majority of medical doctors polled would show it any major concern. A group of honest law enforcement officials should however, move in to investigate the CDC with regards to the creation of false information regarding AIDS and HIV. This is a disease the CDC claims is responsible for approximately 50,000 deaths up until 1992. Yet when there is an autopsy of an AIDS death victim, it is rare you will find HIV. There are also thousands of AIDS cases walking around today world wide, confirmed by the antibody test, with no trace of HIV in them. This is a confirmed fact that the CDC hysterically ignores, and papers like the New York Times never print.

The ABC and CBS networks however, did run specials on this information in late 1993 and early 1994. To no avail, the CDC still stands firm that HIV causes AIDS. A good question to ask any medical professional is, if one is tested positive for HIV antibodies, isn't that a good sign? Those antibodies supposedly are fighting off your AIDS, so the doctor should be happy you have them! Regarding HIV and AIDS, there are thousands of medically diagnosed AIDS cases that have *never* tested positive for HIV. Medical professionals cover their ground on this fact by stating the HIV virus must then be lying dormant, or latent, in the person's body. What a crock! If you, doctor X, have diagnosed Jimmy Y with AIDS, and he is demonstrating classic AIDS symptoms created by the HIV virus, how could that virus be creating the symptoms if it is dormant?!

When you examine the correlation's between AIDS case histories, you realize that the only thing it means to have AIDS is that you are sick and toxic; and usually quite sick and toxic from self induced terrible habits. That's all AIDS is. In the early days of my practice I saw over 100 people who were diagnosed with AIDS, since they heard my nutritional program could save their lives. 90% of them were homosexual men who had a lot of aberrant sex with several partners. I would explain to them how this kind of repeated sexual activity is very draining and toxic to the body, and they would for the most part either slow it down or stop completely. Almost all of them also used recreational drugs on a regular or semi-regular basis. This also had to go. My success rate in treating these patients from 1984 to 1987 was nearly 100%! I am sure if they chose to go on AZT, as their medical doctors screamed for them to do, more than 90% of them would have died. I would venture to say from my professional experience, that most AIDS people die from the poisoning they receive from antiretroviral drugs like AZT.

Burroughs-Welcomb is the top producer of antiretroviral drugs on the market, and they have completed many of their own studies to show that they are quite safe, and that AZT in particular is slowing down the progression of AIDS. The *Concord Institute*, an independent American research organization, came out with quite different results from their study however. They found that 51% of the people using AZT develop lymphatic cancer. Do your own research. Go to the PDR, and look up AZT (it may be found under antiretroviral drugs). Interestingly enough, under side effects of the drug you will find many AIDS symptoms. It is a well known fact in wellness circles today, that those who receive a positive HIV test usually fair well without treatment, assuming they don't kill themselves from the depression and sociological stigma that ensues from ignorance of the facts. Many people who receive an AIDS diagnosis, and use it as an opportunity to heal themselves naturally, excel sometimes even better than they were before the diagnosis! Practically all that receive antiretroviral treatment are either dead or dying. Arthur Ash was totally healthy before he started taking AZT. Kimberly Bourgalis, who sued her dentist in Florida for supposedly infecting her with HIV, had a simple candida yeast infection that was blown into AIDS due to ignorance. She lost about 45 pounds and was eventually confined to a wheel chair from taking AZT.

One of the more frightening sociological aspects of HIV antibody detection, is that one can get completely different answers from two different labs on the same day. Fact is, if you get enough HIV tests, chances are you will eventually wind up positive. This margin of error holds true for most antibody detection blood tests. Further more, in the case of AIDS, to show up positive for HIV means absolutely nothing.

Understand right here and now, that there is no keynote study which proves that HIV causes AIDS. There have been press conferences on this subject that never made it to the major papers. Still, the medical profession will tell people that AIDS is a disease caused by HIV infection, there is no cure and it is extremely fatal.

Another great trick set out by the CDC regarding AIDS, came in 1987 when they changed the diseases' diagnostic parameters. After this date, the following diseases can also be diagnosed as AIDS: candida infection, cervical cancer of the uterus, herpes simplex disorders, malignant lymphomas, encephalopathy, dementia, weight loss or mal nutrition, heart attacks, strokes, cirrhosis of the liver, salmonella infection, TB, and my favorite, *suicide!* These parameters are way our of control, and resemble more of a comedy routine sooner than science.

Chapter Eight
Good-bye Germ Theory

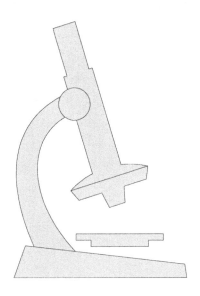

When we talk about the germ theory, we enter into a realm of historical debate long forgotten in America. To date, there is still no logical basis in science for the germ theory, however it has become fundamental law with concern to the medical profession, and the pharmaceutical companies which support it.

In a very real sense, the *"science"* of medicine is more like a dogmatic religion, preaching eternal damnation to non-believers and excommunication (in the form of de-licensing and jail) for non-conformists. The ultimate demons in this religion are the *"germs,"* a group of fiendish opportunists who attack and take advantage of otherwise *good and wholesome God lovin folks*. You are defenseless against these devils unless you pray with the high priests of medicine, who act as an intermediary between you and God. If you pray with them hard enough, maybe God will help you. Most likely not however, since the art of praying for a cure with the medical profession statistically looks worse and worse each year. With concern to malignant cancer, the AMA has established 5 year survival rate guidelines for doctors since that is usually how long the average patient endures before death. Is has been shown statistically however, that if you do not follow medical treatment for a malignant diagnosis, and if you choose to do nothing with your cancer, not even change your style of life and diet, on average you will live 12 years. This value can obviously be improved past the 12 year mark with proper life changes in diet and detoxification. Far better than your survival odds look while choosing to stay with the standard medical approach of radiation and chemotherapy. Your odds look pretty grim within the medical faith. Thomas Szasz, MD had this to say about the religion of medicine in *Reason* magazine in June of 1998:

"Using the coercive apparatus of the State to force people to submit to the ministrations of doctors of medicine is a persecution in the name of health, exactly as using the coercive apparatus of the State to force people to submit to the ministrations of doctors of divinity was persecution in the name of God."

The idea of entities called "germs" maybe causing disease predates *Louis Pasteur by* several centuries. However, in 1878 Louis Pasteur was credited with the full tenets of the germ theory, solidifying all its' laws and postulates which are used this very day in the determination of disease. History paints a much better picture of Pasteur than reality dictates, as he is credited with solving the mystery of fermentation, the silk worm disease in France, the rabies dilemma of his time, as well as being able to control the spread of *anthrax* through his vaccine. Hey, after all, its' been on TV! It must have happened that way.

Who was Louis Pasteur, really? He was a chemist. He had no formal training in biology, as the story dictates. The discovery of fermentation did not belong to Pasteur alone. The Silk Worm "cure" that he instituted cut the production of silk in France by half. More people got sick and died from his rabies vaccine then ever had rabies to begin with during his time. In 1956, JAMA (The Journal of the American Medical Association) reported that the Academy of Medicine in France found *"Pasteur's rabies vaccinations may be followed as much as 20 years later with a rare form of psychosis."* This, at the very least, shows the AMA acknowledged at some point in time that vaccines can cause health problems decades later. It has been shown statistically that in countries where the Pasteur rabies vaccine has been employed, the number of deaths from hydrophobia (rabies) *has actually increased and not diminished.* Pasteur's anthrax vaccine in Russia was nothing short of a disaster. 4,500 sheep were administered the vaccine, and 3,600 dropped dead almost immediately following. Pasteur's rabies vaccine killed King Alexander of Greece, who was given the treatment after being bitten by a monkey. He died within one week of the vaccine. These are all the wonderful Pasteurian facts you've never heard in school.

What really happened around 1878? Well, it turns out that
the real credit for most of Pasteur's success belonged to a man
named *Pierre Bechamp*. He was a French scientist contemporary to
Pasteur, who for some reason not fully understood, made all the
discoveries given claim to Pasteur well before they became common
knowledge. Pasteur and Bechamp may have had some form of
working agreement that was never known to historians, but it is
said in some historical circles that Pasteur actually plagiarized most
of Bechamp's hard work. Bechamp was known as a quiet, humble
man that did not like the limelight. Bechamp continued to pursue
his work quietly as Pasteur became more popular with most of
Bechamp's earliest discoveries, including fermentation.

Bechamp's work was based on the observation of live tissues (as
opposed to dead tissue samples of lab work today). In these live
tissues, he saw tiny bodies he called *Microzyma*. He then went on to
propose publicly that these Microzyma were the basic unit of life,
indestructible, immutable and eternal. He found these bodies in
both plant and animal tissue. He found them in both healthy and
diseased tissue. In healthy tissue, he found them to be normal,
constructive parts of the growing metabolism of the cell. In unhealthy
tissue, *he discovered that they evolved into bacteria*. By this time,
Pasteur was off on his own running with his recreation of the germ
theory. He did not realize what Bechamp had realized; *that the
medium determines whether or not micro-organisms, such as bacteria,
are present*. Bechamp saw clearly that bacteria are endogenous; that
is, they come from within us. From within our own tissues and cells
from some basic point of life, in which he called Microzyma. The
important difference here, is that Bechamp realized bacteria and
other microbes are formed out of necessity by the body itself. They
do not come from some outside attacking mode of virulence. It's too
bad that Pasteur, who was best at promoting himself, did not catch
on to this theory of the Microzyma. For if he did, things would be a
lot better today for it.

Bechamp carried on some fantastic experiments that never made
it to the history books. All of his work confirmed his belief in the
presence of Microzyma, that all bacteria originate from them, and

that bacteria are pleomorphic (able to change shape) upon the need of the tissue. Pasteur on the other hand, claimed that bacteria are monomorphic (only one shape per strain, or "species" of bacteria), and that they originate from outside the body in nature. Pasteur postulated that there is one bacteria or other microbe for each disease. This microbe is the causative agent of the disease, and you will find it in every sick tissue of that diseased person or animal.

Bechamp obtained the carcass of a kitten and embedded it in calcium carbonate (chalk) for approximately 8 years. He took special care to prepare the carcass aseptically, which means no "germs" could possibly get in through the outside world. Upon examination of the carcass after this 8 year period, as would be suspected he found it primarily decomposed. He repeated this experiment again, only this time he removed all the dead internal organs, treated them separately with another aseptic process, and examined the organs and the skeleton separately after a shorter period of years. He found identical results; in both cases, there were varying forms of bacteria with abundant Microzyma. Other scientists became intrigued with Bechamp's work and decided to repeat the process for themselves. Internal organs were taken from varying dead animals. The external portions of the organs were then treated aseptically, usually with an alcohol base or other antiseptic, bactericidal fluid. This was to ensure that no external microbes could affect the experiment. Some of these organs were even left suspended in a constant stream of bactericide. In all cases, it was found that where the antiseptic fluid could not reach, endogenous microbial activity flourished. How did these microbes get inside the organ? A doctor today may tell you that of course certain strains of bacteria and microbes are endogenous. They sit inside our body, in all our organs, waiting to take advantage of the medium when its' resistance is low, or in this case, quite dead, to take over and ingest the now morbid organic matter.

The medical profession is mostly correct with this fact, but they miss one subtle and very vital point. The microbes, such as the differing strains of bacteria, are not there as evil opportunists; hidden time bombs just waiting in the shadows to take advantage of our low resistance. They are actually created out of our necessity, following the commands of the organic web of life. They spring forth within each cell upon the need. In a living person, they spring forth to eat poisonous organic material, with the most common form being that of foreign or excess proteins, in an effort to cleanse the system. If there is an abundance of toxicity, especially in the form of proteins either from vaccines or poor dietary habits, they will be created in abundance. Their respiratory, metabolic and excretory processes (breathing, eating and going to the bathroom processes, just like you and I), can then make the surrounding body tissue sore. This is when we go to the medical doctor, he takes a culture of our throat and tells us we have a bacterial infestation. Here, take these antibiotics! This is as smart as blaming rats for the garbage pileups that occur during a sanitation worker strike. The rats are just there doing their job! They eat garbage, and if you don't want to see them around your neighborhood anymore, well then, clean up the garbage. Spraying rat poison on the garbage pileups is only a temporary solution, and one that has serious side effects to the greater good of your neighborhood.

Taking antibiotics for this kind of bacterial "infection," is the same bad idea. The bacteria did not create your sickness. Nor did the virus, the yeast, or any other natural microbe you can name (save the ones created by government genetic experiments to actually cause havoc with living tissue). You are sick because you have a sick system, either physically, emotionally, spiritually, or some combination of the three. The microbes that arise from your cells, quite possibly through Bechamp's Microzyma, are members of the web of life called *Saprophytes*. These are defined as a group of micro-organisms whose sole existence is designed by God to break down dead, diseased and or dying organic material into its' simpler forms of organic chemicals. The Biblical ashes to ashes and dust to dust scenario. Nothing in the web of life is ever wasted. When physical matter becomes devoid of life force; i.e., when you leave your physical body at the time of so called "death," the organic materials which comprise the physical form are broken down and thus returned to the Earth from whence they arose. The physical form cannot survive without the spirit, life force energy which animates it through the nervous system. It is simply a vehicle for this energy, which as Einstein stated, "can never be created nor destroyed."

Now consider a smaller version of total physical death; simple cellular death, which occurs thousands of times each second with the rebirth of new, healthy body cells. In a totally fit and healthy individual, white blood cells of the immune system find it easy to handle the job of cleaning up these dead cells with some help from indigenously created microbes, like bacteria. This is precisely why, healthy or not, a *throat culture will always show some bacterial activity*. Microbes are *never absent* from your body. They are a ubiquitous form, and fact of life. But most people are not so healthy, since most people do not exercise healthy habits, physically, emotionally and spiritually. To the direct proportional degree that we do not exercise healthy habits, we have a proportional level of increased cellular death. When the white blood cells and antibodies of the immune system cannot handle the load of this increased cellular clean up, microbes are created, indigenously, as extra workers for the process.

Pasteur, being the chemist that he was, saw this connection (which he most likely acquired from Bechamp) that bacteria and other microbes carry out chemical processes within the body. He also noticed that these chemical processes have to do with microbial respiration, metabolism and excretion. Pasteur's difference however was in his lack of vision. The party line during his time was demanding a culprit enemy for the high level of disease in certain areas of the globe, and Pasteur was determined to give them one. Microbes, due to Pasteur, then became the phantom *ghosts* of disease. A new enemy to wage war on, taking the responsibility (once again) off the people; in this case it meant the responsibility of providing sanitary living conditions, both externally and internally.

As an example, during the time of the so called *"bubonic plague,"* the living conditions in France and most other areas of Europe were far from ideal for the bulk of citizens. There was no sanitation in larger, more congested areas of city life, where people crammed together in small living quarters would dump their feces and urine onto the streets. The most popular food of the average commoner was *lard pie.* You read that correctly; that's the same as *FAT PIE!* These fat pies were usually mixed with potatoes and other heavy starches. Another contribution to the generalized poisoning of Europe of that time was cooking with *LEAD* utensils. You can only imagine how a diet of this nature, prepared with lead utensils, would clog up the circulatory system with accumulated fat and poisons. Was there any doubt that these people would develop large, painful buboes glands (hence the *bubonic* plague). The treatment for the bubonic plague was similar to the intent of modern day chemotherapy; i.e., cut out what appears to be the bad parts. So people had their glands removed from their arm pits and groin. Now as you most likely are aware, the glands of the body belong to the *lymphatic* system. This system cleanses the blood, with the glands around the neck, arm pit and groin acting as filters. These people lived in highly toxic circumstances most of their lives, and now their swollen and overworked blood filters were being removed. Not too smart, but then again, its medicine. Medical philosophy has not changed much in 500 years, centering itself around either *cutting* something out or *drugging* something out. The party line on the bubonic plague, which is hysterically still taught as such, is that rats carried fleas which carried microbes that created the disease. This is total nonsense.

External sanitation improved by leaps and bounds into the turn of the 20th century. This is why all statistical research shows major infectious disease rates declining rapidly around 1910. But the war on germs was seen to be a worthwhile one, most likely due to a mixture of human superstition and greed. Out of this war was born the oppressive medical cartel we are all struggling with today. It's time we educate the people as to the truth, and real purpose of these microbes, and end this fictional war. It is high time to say, "Good-Bye Germ Theory!"

The Bechamp experiment was reproduced many times by many scientists through the early 1900's. Upon the advancement of laboratory procedure, isolated tissues were used instead of entire organs suspended in aseptic fluid. The same results were produced time and time again. On the outside of the tissue that had been in contact with the aseptic material, there were obviously no microbes. There were microbes, as before, within all of the more internal cells that did not contact the fluid. Finally around the turn of the 20th century, there were some interesting technological advances which gave birth to the work of another brilliant American scientist named Raymond Riffe.

In the 1920's, Riffe postulated that there was something he was not seeing when he looked at cellular materials under the common compound microscope of his time. He brilliantly theorized that the reason he could not see everything one could see when viewing living tissue under a microscope, was because of the lack of *ultraviolet light*, in which the common microscope's lenses could not detect. The glass of a common microscope does not allow UV radiation to enter the field of view. Riffe then built a series of amazing microscopes, that still to this day are second to none. For example, all of his lenses were made of quartz crystal, and not glass. This allowed the full range of UV light to come into the scope's field of view. He then began to see another realm of existence.

Riffe also came up with a system of magnification that rivaled early electron microscopes of our day; about 150,000 X magnification. He viewed all kinds of tissues with his new scopes, live and dead, and found Bechamp's Microzyma everywhere. When viewing these Microzyma with the quartz scope, under higher and higher magnification he found smaller and smaller units of Microzyma. Like Bechamp, Riffe discovered that these small units of life spontaneously evolved into varying forms of larger micro-organisms, solely dependent on the type of tissue in which they existed (healthy or toxic). Amazingly enough, he completed experiments where through carefully controlling the level of toxicity within any given tissue, *he was able to have the Microzyma evolve into a viral type of organism that created cancer in the tissue every time.* This of course, indicated an intimate connection between cellular toxicity and cancer. From this place, he attempted to work on a cure for cancer by reversing the process. These experiments were not successful, however Riffe continued his work to the discovery of healing EMF (electromagnetic fields). He built a device which created EMF's that could disintegrate certain viral substances from a distance. Riffe was truly a brilliant man, unfortunately lost to history on purpose through the actions of the medical cartel.

The Journal for the Franklin Institute in Pennsylvania wrote an article about Riffe's work in 1944. The title of the article was, *"The New Microscopes:"*

"Riffe showed that by altering the environment and food supply, friendly germs such as colon bacillus can be converted into pathogenic germs, such as typhoid, and that this process is reversible. Experiments in the Riffe lab established that the virus of cancer, like viruses from other diseases, can easily be changed from one form to another by means of altering the media upon which they feed . . . . with the first change of the media, the cancer virus becomes enlarged (looking very much like E. coli) . . . . observation under an ordinary scope is made possible through a second alteration in media . . . . a third change is undergone upon an asparagus based media, where this cancer virus is now transformed from its' filterable state into cryptomyces pleomorphia fungi . . . ."

This is a very important article to the nature of our discussion. Riffe was able to show from this experiment, that took place in the 1940's, that he could take the virus that created cancer in his lab animals and turn it into E. Coli (the friendly colon bacillus), and then into a fungus! This fits in well with the basic premise of our text. These microbes are saprophytes, produced primarily for breaking down matter into its' constituent elements. This is precisely what they do when you get sick. They are not attacking you. Indeed, they are attempting to help bring you back to better health and wholeness. By removing the diseased, toxic cellular material from your tissues, you are better able to create new healthy cells to heal the tissue. *The nature of disease is NOT germs. The true nature of disease is the toxic input you place into your body, or randomly run across in your drinking water from pollution or radiation, and your body's quest to eliminate it.*

We said before that so called "germs" are ubiquitous. They are ever present, in many varying forms in both healthy and sick people. These microbes kick into what modern scientists call *pathogens*, when the media is toxic and conducive to clean up. When you enter into a healing crisis, and your body is throwing off toxins, these "germs" appear out of your very substance, to help eliminate, process and break down these toxins. *Germs have absolutely no causal relationship to disease.* But germs do appear to help you clean out, because put quite simply, *your disease is your cure!* Modern medical professionals have made a very false, yet understandable assumption, that germs create disease due to their mere presence in sick people. This is a vast oversimplification of the real process however, and it is high time to end it.

Riffe's work is actually preceded by another great study completed by Dr. H. Rosenaeu at the Mayo Biological Laboratory in 1910. He did the reverse process of Riffe, who showed you can turn bacteria into different forms by altering their environment. Roseneau took a myriad of disease germs and placed them in the same media, and found that over time they all transformed into the same micro-organism!

Rational Bacteriology is a milestone, yet out of print text of microbiology. It was independently published in 1953 by three doctors, Verner, Weiant and Watkins. This text confirms Bechamp's work, and speaks of the actual basis of bacteriology that is not Pasteurian propaganda. It cites countless experiments, hidden from the public, which prove that micro-organisms like bacteria are formed from "granules" which are inherent as a healthy constituent of every living cell.

When these granules morph into bacteria, they do so to *ACTUALLY BOOST IMMUNITY AND AID IN THE HEALING PROCESS. Staphylococci bacteria were found to be a primary force involved in the production of white blood cells for immunity against varying poisons, as well as generalized blood clotting.* This truth is miles away from the Pasteurian nonsense we were all led to believe in school; that these *"bad germs"* are single minded opportunists that work for your persistent demise. Nothing could be further from the truth. They are part of the bodies defense mechanism to clean house and purify the system back to homeostasis (balance). They exist in this granular form until needed. When are they needed? When your body has reached a certain limit of toxicity from your external environment, or more likely, your dietary and drinking habits. What does the medical establishment say to do once they detect these bacterial healing agents? Wipe them out with antibiotics (translation is "against-life")and other toxic drugs, and further turn your internal body fluids into a toxic soup. This Germ-Theory of the Dark Ages is nothing but a deliberate mass insanity pushed upon society to gain profit and power. By acting against microbes as the medical establishment dictates, one is actually helping to dig one's own grave, while paying someone else to show where to dig. This insanity must end.

Rational Bacteriology states:

"Extensive studies of bacteria show definitely that there are no fixed species. A cocci can become a bacilli, a spirili, and vice versa. Streptococci and pneumococci interchange. All bacteria either acquire or loose virulence depending upon their environment. Bacteria change to molds and vice versa in response to adequate environmental stimuli. Furthermore, they can resolve into their smallest form, a sub-microscopic granule [Bechamp's Microzyma]. The bacterial "toxins" which were once thought to be entirely free of particles, are not really homogeneous solutions at all, but actually contain the tiny granular stages of bacteria which broke down to form them."

The largest problem I have discovered with presenting such evidence in today's "modern scientific world," is that the professionals say, "so what if all this is true! They can transform all they like, and who cares about Microzyma? Germs still cause disease!" Studies are not done on the correlation of "germs" to disease anymore, because the scientific community assumes that germs create disease without question. This is similar to the witch hunts of old, where everyone was certain there were witches running about, and if you were a non-believer, perhaps you should be burned at the stake as well! Any work challenging the correlation of germs to any disease is simply not supported, and due to finances, simply viewed as a waste of time and money. What pharmaceutical company do you know that will fund a study to prove that germs have no correlation with the creation of disease? Bechamp's findings can easily be reproduced today, but no one wants to reproduce them. The medical cartel has suppressed any information available on such discoveries, and financially discourages medical professionals from inquiring further study into Microzyma. Since virtually no one on Earth knows of this information today, it can be said that they have been immensely successful in their suppression of the truth.

> *Party Line #11*: Koch's postulates are the indisputable proof that germs cause disease. They are the foundation stone of proof for the germ theory.

Junior doctors and to be medical professionals, from most health professions, learn this party line about *Koch's Postulates*. It is perhaps, one of the most embarrassing facts of so called "modern science," that these postulates prevail as the foundation stone for medical diagnosis. The postulates, in and of themselves, are not invalid. They are quite scientific. However, what we are not told is that *not one single disease of recorded history can be explained by using them as a guideline. Not one.* If anything, Koch's postulates can be very effective in proving just the opposite! That so called "germs" have absolutely nothing to do with the creation of disease. With concern to any given disease process, any high school biology student could adequately dispute any one of these postulates, with mere common biological knowledge. These postulates come to us from the famous German bacteriologist Robert Koch, who won a Nobel Prize for their development in 1905. For the purpose of saying Good-Bye to the germ theory, lets consider them in some detail.

Koch's Postulates

1. In order for a germ to cause disease, the germ has to be found in every case of the disease.
2. In order for a germ to cause disease, it can never be found apart from the disease.
3. In order for a germ to cause disease, it must be capable of disease culture outside the body.
4. In order for a germ to cause disease, it must be capable of producing by injection the same disease as that undergone by the body from which it was taken (the basis of vaccines).

Any honest mainstream bacteriologist will tell you each of these postulates are completely fictitious with concern to the correlation of germs and disease. Let's take each one separately.

1. *Found in every case of the disease.* Hey, you mean just like AIDS! HIV is proven to be doing absolutely nothing in healthy people, and again, thousands of medically diagnosed AIDS cased have shown up with no trace of HIV (see chapter 6). It is historical fact that you can go through case after case after case, finding people being diagnosed with various diseases while being unable to locate the germ. *WHERE'S THE GERM*!? How do medical professionals find many of these "germs" anyway? Through antibody tests that don't mean anything, and as we have discussed, are highly unreliable. Even if a specific "pathogen" is found in a sick person, there is no way to prove a solid, causal relationship.

A 1993 national television special featured *"what is the real cause of AIDS?"* This program told the truth in a way I've never seen before on mainstream television, and I commend the powers that be who delivered this information to the public nationally. It is only through the efforts of good people like these *"in the know,"* that the public can be saved from the parasitic nature of the medical cartel. It is because of efforts like this one to expose medical fraud, that we as a nation of people were saved from a massive *"AIDS Epidemic"* scam masterminded by the CDC and EIS (for more information on the EIS, please see next chapter). I would like to take some time here in the consideration of this first postulate to reproduce some quotes from that show, since they are most relevant to our discussion.

The show began by stating that HIV and AIDS have no proven correlation. It then switched to *"the man with the deep pockets in the AIDS establishment,"* Dr. Anthony Fauchi, director of the *National Institute of Allergy and Infectious Diseases.* Dr. Fauchi had this to say:

> *"What's next is to develop and appropriate, safe and effective therapy, and a safe and effective vaccine. That's the bottom line of it. You have a disease, you identify the cause, you identify a treatment, and you get a vaccine for it."*

Find the bug. Study the bug. Kill the bug. Teach your body how to kill the bug. This guy is a standard medical cartel employee. I have a list in my possession of the 1991 membership of the EIS, and guess what! It shouldn't surprise you that Dr. Anthony Fauchi is a member. Dr. Robert Gallo, probably one of the loudest mouths of the government and AIDS establishment screaming that HIV causes AIDS, is also a member. It shouldn't surprise you that none of the other doctors quoted here, who state just the opposite of Drs. Fauchi and Gallo, are members.

Dr. Luc Montagnier was the first to isolate and study HIV in Europe. He had this to say:

> *"I think people should really think and perhaps try to have new concepts, because AIDS is a complicated disease and not caused only by HIV."*

Dr. Walter Gilbert, a Nobel prize winner in microbiology at Harvard University had this to say:

"The major thing that concerns me by calling HIV the cause of AIDS is that we do not have a proof of causation. This is a major reason to be concerned. The crucial parts of this argument are that all cases of AIDS are not associated with the virus, and there is an inference made that all people with the virus will ultimately come down with AIDS. This is of course not known to be a fact."

The interviewer asked Dr. Joseph Sonnebend, a private AIDS researcher and clinician, that if HIV does not cause AIDS, why does it say it does in popular medical texts of microbiology that medical students learn from? The doctor answered:

"It is most definitely not a fact that HIV causes AIDS. That is a conjecture, and not an established fact. The harm in the whole notion of a speculation presented as fact, such as this one, is that if the speculation proves to be untrue in the long run, this means that research and work on whatever is truly going on has been neglected. This of course with a disease like AIDS can be translated into the loss of tens of thousands of lives."

Dr. Robert Root-Bernstein is a physiologist at Michigan State University, and author of the book, *"Rethinking AIDS."* He had this to say:

"When I look at AIDS patients, I can find that no one who develops AIDS that does not have a multitude of immunosuppressant agents working on them simultaneously. The logic of the war on AIDS is seriously flawed."

The interviewer asked Dr. Root-Bernstein what would happen if you injected or otherwise exposed a totally healthy person to the HIV virus. He answered:

"Actually, you don't need to propose an experiment such as this, it has already been done. There are people who are married to blood transfusion patients, people who are married to

*hemophiliacs, who have been exposed to HIV from these means.
There are surgeons who cut themselves all the time while working
on AIDS patients, and these people are free of HIV. Even more
interesting are the several dozen cases in the medical records
where people have demonstrated that healthy individuals with no
other known risks, have developed an infection through one of
these routes. They can show the HIV was in their blood stream,
and that it infected some of their cells, and they developed
antibodies to it, and that at a later time, they could no longer
find any HIV. In some cases, these people even lost their
antibodies to HIV, and all have remained perfectly healthy."*

Dr. Anthony Fauchi had a scripted answer to these doctors:

*"There can be a long process that it takes for the immune system to
go down after infection with HIV. People are very different. Some
people have a response to the virus that the immune decline is very
rapid. Some people take a longer period of time to get sick."*

Hmmmmmmm? Doesn't this mean that the *real causes* of AIDS
are those factors which cause one person to have a rapid decline,
and others to have a "slow decline." Dr. Fauchi simply routes the
medical party line that if infected, *you must* be sick at some time,
and therefore, you are sick now! This is like saying that because I
burned myself with the Iron last Tuesday, next time I use the iron
I will again burn myself. Dr. Fauchi's statements on the show were
nothing short of an admission that HIV has no scientific correlation
to AIDS.

Dr. Peter Duesberg is a hero for the people regarding this AIDS
epidemic fraud. He is a pioneering virologist at the University of
California at Berkley, and has for years been the loudest voice stating
that HIV and AIDS have nothing to do with one another. He said:

*"I would drink HIV infested water all day long. There would be
absolutely no risk in doing so. There is no proof that HIV causes
AIDS. In addition, I am familiar with retroviruses, how they*

behave and what they do, and on those counts I am confident enough that HIV, no matter how, couldn't possibly cause AIDS. Because of this view, my funding for viral research was not renewed. But there is a growing number of people who are asking questions. Another thing, is that this is just the tip of the iceberg. Many people who have doubts that I know of tell me that they can't afford to speak up now because their research plans and grant money depend on HIV. If I join you, my grants will be terminated just like yours."

The interviewer asked Dr. Root-Bernstein the following:

"I have a grant to look at something which you and I both agree is silly, but neither of us are going to say anything about it since it's primarily about receiving the money."

Dr. Root-Bernstein responded:

"To put it bluntly, that is a good statement, yes."

Despite everything you've just read, Dr. Fauchi still stated:

"Certainly the amount of funding to HIV is clearly greater than the funding going into other areas, and for very logical reasons. The logical reason is, that if you don't have the virus, you don't get sick."

Dr. Fauchi seriously needs to step out of his office at the National Institute of Allergy and Infectious Diseases and read what the research proves. HIV clearly contradicts all of Koch's postulates, and cannot possibly be a prime causative factor in the development of AIDS.

By chasing HIV, Dr. Fauchi and the government have spent over 4 billion dollars in HIV research. A very small percentage is devoted to studying other factors besides HIV. The amount of funding for research that examines if HIV has nothing to do with

AIDS, is 0%. So well over 4 billion dollars has been spent on examining an AIDS culprit that doesn't hurt any cells, and that when it supposedly kills someone you are unable to locate it. It is the hallmark of a poorly positioned hypothesis that it produces no results in research, and HIV research is the poster example of such a dilemma.

Dr. Walter Gilbert remembered when the EIS attempted to make cancer an infectious disease, caused by a virus. He said:

> *"This comes out of a disappointed war on cancer. This is the political force which has turned into the war on HIV and AIDS. By pointing to a viral causation, you can attempt to promise people that science would do something about it in the short run."*

This is a very nice way to view the situation. It assumes that at least the government is trying to find answers for the people. The truth is however, that the medical cartel has promulgated the AIDS epidemic for profit, and that is a statement very few people are willing to admit, but I surmise many agree with.

Continuing on with our discussion of Koch's postulates;

#2) *Never found apart from the disease.* Another laugh. In a relatively short time after Koch came up with this postulate, it was realized to be an immense error with concern to micro-organisms. During any study on any day of the year, it can be shown that healthy people are teaming with varying forms of bacteria, viruses, yeast and fungi for many communicable diseases. How come these people are without symptoms and are otherwise, healthy?

#3) *Capable of culture outside the body.* Guess what? Any medical professional knows you cannot grow bacteria or virus on healthy tissue. When you attempt to grow an AIDS culture of HIV virus on healthy tissue, the T-Lymphocyte count (major white blood cell) does not get damaged. In fact, it shoots up! Isn't the AIDS virus supposed to destroy white blood cells upon contact? A researcher will never be able to grow bacteria or viruses on healthy tissue. Of course, you can culture any kind of bacteria or other microbe outside the body. But what are you using to do such a thing? Beef broth. Albumin based broth. Eggs. What do all these things have in common? They're all dead! They're all morbid organic matter. Just the food saprophytes love. Microbes look for this morbid organic matter in your body as well.

#4) *Capable of producing by injection the same disease, as that undergone by the body from which it was taken.* In February of 1921, a U.S. government bulletin reported that the *hygienic laboratory #123* did a study, where they tried in every possible way to contaminate 62 Navy personnel with influenza. They took sputum from influenza cases, and sprayed it down their throats (YUK!). They sprayed the same on their foods. They kept these people in constant contact with influenza patients. The conclusion of the study showed "no appreciable reactions."

Don't we all experience aspects of this study on a daily basis? How many people do you come into contact with, in which you don't catch anything from? Why is it that many people don't get the flu each year? How come what they do is not studied? These are very good questions that we must push our lawmakers to take seriously.

Chapter Nine
Spontaneous Generation

This hypothesis of pathogenesis or infection stemming from some microbe has very clearly not supported society since the time of it's inception with Louis Pasteur. It has certainly supported the varying medical businesses in ultra profitable ways, centered around the pharmaceutical companies, which rely on people believing in infection and pathogenic organisms that anyone can simply "catch" from someone else or the "outside" environment; but in reality this way of thinking has not supported the *people* of the planet in any positive way. This theory of germ infection and pathogenesis has accomplished a control of the planets' laws, values and mores which the medical establishment and pharmaceutical companies spend a ton of time and energy in promoting.

This is of course, all at the expense of the people, since this way of believing and thinking keeps them sick, whether or not they are manifesting symptoms. The bulk of the planet believes that they can be invaded by a microbe which can bring them from a state of complete health to complete disease, simply by a matter of exposure. While in many cases this scenario is true when considering *parasites*, it is complete nonsense when speaking of micro-organisms considered to be "*germs.*" By their very definition, a parasite is an opportunistic and quite large organism, single or multi celled, that *attacks* the body using it for its' own gain while giving you nothing in return. This is hardly the case with micro-organisms, which exist in a commensalistic relationship with the Human organism; i.e., they exist within your body as a natural component and play an important role in the homeostasis of your being.

Has any doctor or teacher ever told you this fact? Can you imagine what would happen to the medical profession and the pharmaceutical companies if people suddenly became empowered enough to listen to their intuition on this matter? These present *disease care* establishments need a constant supply of diseased people to maintain their extreme power and wealth. If the bulk of society were to stop and realize for even a moment that *they are in charge of their own personal state of health, and that the healing and health maintenance ability of the body is well within their reach,* the medical profession would cease to exist and the pharmaceutical companies would go out of business.

All that is required here is a small shift in consciousness; one that brings people away from the stance of helpless victim to empowered Human. To say that any new theory that challenges the Germ Theory needs to be fully researched before consideration is absurd. Statistics tell all! Just look at the state of health of the average American citizen, and this is all the proof you need. Disease runs rampant in America, and absolute health is indeed the rarity. This is all due to the attitude, and aptitude, of victim consciousness and irresponsibility for how we live our lives, which is truly what is keeping people sick.

This germ, infective and pathogenic hypothesis simply does not work when considering any stream of logic. Therefore, we need a paradigm shift to get out of the pickle we are in as a species. This involves the more responsible and logical hypothesis first proposed by Pierre Bechamp just before the rise of Pasteurian thought and popularity. Bechamps' research documented small bodies which were healthy and natural components of every living cell, and he called them *Microzyma*. These Microzyma are smaller than even the smallest of cellular organelles, and need a special brand of dark field and ultraviolet sensitive microscopes to be seen. Once examined, they are witnessed to be completely *pleomorphic*, which simply means they are able to change shape when ever they please. In effect, they are *shape shifters,* and what causes them to change shape? Simply the nature of the environment in which they exist.

Around the time of Charles Darwin, this school of thought was called *Spontaneous Generation,* which was a very popular school of scientific consideration. The thought was that due to the nature of the environment, energy over time naturally would shift the DNA of any given animal or plant species, thus creating more favorable physical characteristics for survival in future generations. The Giraffe was once a short necked animal, and the stress which was created on its' neck from the persistent stretching upward to reach an ample food supply of leaves, created a shift in its' DNA collectively as a species which brought about the need for a longer neck; hence the long neck Giraffes we see today. Darwin challenged this popular thought by proposing an idea of *the survival of the fittest*. Taking the same example, he suggested that natural DNA varieties of short and long necked Giraffes once co-existed together, however the short necked variety became extinct through a lack of ample food supply. The long necked variety however overcame this problem by their ability to reach more leaves, and thus were stronger and faster to avoid carnivorous predators. In the long run, we have witnessed that Darwin's theories of evolution have gained momentum over the years, whereas spontaneous generation has been left behind. With concern to this issue of evolution I believe that both theories have relevance.

But the idea of spontaneous generation was not left behind by Pierre Bechamp. Especially after his discovery of Microzyma, he theorized that within the microscopic world spontaneous generation occurs far more rapidly than in the gross, physical world. He witnessed these Microzyma change shape at the earliest sign of an environmental shift, and he further theorized that this shift occurs as a balancing mechanism of some important homeostasis processes undergone by the individual cell. In fact, these Microzyma are so pleomorphic that Bechamp witnessed them change into virtually every viral, bacterial and fungal microbial shape known to science, simply by shifting the environment in which they existed.

The medical establishment filters this process through the germ theory, insisting these organisms are monomorphic, arriving on the scene from some unseen place, and invading the body for some opportunistic reason. The medical establishment then uses their brand of junk science to classify and categorize these varying forms of Microzyma, which freezes them in time as the villains of disease creation. They swab a red and sore throat of a child and take a culture, only to find an abundance of streptococcus pyogenes. But they are only looking at a single snapshot, taken out of context of a vastly abundant process! If they were to take the right measures in science and dive deeper into the study of those organisms, they would see the bigger picture; the entire movie! They would witness these streptococci change as the child's diet, or other unhealthy habits which precipitated the red and sore throat in the first place, did indeed change.

This theory laid out for us by Bechamp holds tremendous potential for the well being of our planet here and now. It shows us that if we are responsible for our lives; if we manage our diets in a healthy fashion which is consistent with our species; if we maintain our fluid balance properly to persistently cleanse our circulatory system and lymphatic system; if we strive to keep our circulatory and lymphatic systems alkaline; if we take more action to think and emote more positively, productively and responsibly, then Microzyma will have no need to change into the so called *pathogenic and infective microbes* as they are classified by medicine.

Clearly, the problem is not the microbe. The problem is the individual lifestyle which creates an environmental need for the production of virus, bacteria and fungus through spontaneous generation from Microzyma. These living things are not the opportunistic villains they are made out to be. They are a very methodical class of living organisms called *Saprophytes.* Saprophytes have one major job on the planet, and that is simply to *ingest dead organic matter.* When an animal or plant dies and falls onto the Earth, these organisms rise up to the occasion and eat the now dead organic matter that has become void of life force, or nerve energy. They rise up within each cell of the human body to accomplish the same task. In our present society, the average person is replete with excess proteinaceous waste and other dietary toxins that can be eliminated with more responsible eating habits. Microzyma persistently change into the necessary Saprophytic forms, and seem ubiquitous in most folks, since they are always on call to eat an endless supply of dead organic waste in the form of clumpy undigested proteins which are abundant in the average individual. This of course, leads to another problem of excess metabolic waste production from the ongoing Saprophytic activity within the body, which in and of itself kills more cells through the toxicity it generates. When a medical professional notices a so called *pathogen* creating toxins in and around the cells through their metabolic processes, they believe they are attacking the person, when in fact they are simply there doing their job in an attempt to purify the person by eating the dead organic material which is foreign and highly toxic to the body. Once again, the doctor needs to look at the entire movie instead of a single photo taken out of context.

Clearly, this Pasteurian way of thinking; this *theory* everything is based on called the *Germ Theory*, has done nothing to productively serve society. Logically we thus have to look to a more common sense philosophy like spontaneous generation, backed up by Bechamps' research. Even more clearly, not one sentence of medical cartel *"research"* which supports the germ theory can refute the validity of spontaneous generation. Regarding every single piece of propaganda research insisting on microbial pathogenic infection which attacks people, we can say, *"Now wait just a minute!" There is no evidence now, and never has been any evidence, that these micro-organisms are solely responsible for this disease process!*

Germ theory research relies on the supposition, or more poignantly the *superstition,* that just because we see these micro-organisms present at the scene of the crime in whatever numbers within a sick person, that they are the cause of the disease and difficulty. This is the same reasoning which would lead one to believe that rats create garbage. NO! The rats don't create the garbage on the streets! We create it! The rats are just there doing their job, because the garbage is sitting on the street way too long, especially during a sanitation strike. ***Throughout history, what most people believe were epidemics created by infection through micro-organisms, were in reality issues of both external and internal sanitation.*** But many parents say, *"hey wait a minute! My kid gets sick through the contagious pattern at her primary school. Once almost* *half the class and the teacher were out because they passed the same bug amongst themselves for weeks!* This is not true however. They passed nothing between themselves; in fact, they were more likely reacting collectively to the toxicity which runs rampant in most primary schools from mold and other fungus spores, as well as different chemical toxins. Children are more susceptible to these things in the cold weather. These things occur from a stance of group detoxification, which also has energetic components which can certainly influence people who are in close contact on a daily basis. The Human body's energy fields are more powerful than most people can even imagine. When one Human body is detoxing, an almost magnetic effect radiates out from such individuals causing the same purifying effects in the immediate environment of people around them. We are not witnessing epidemics or contagious infections; we are witnessing a group healing process which is totally natural to our species.

The next logical area of discussion after knowing this information on spontaneous generation and how all things have purpose, is the benefit of allowing yourself and your child to experience an acute illness from the get go through to it's natural, healthy completion. This is God's way of creating a natural lifetime immunity which leads to a healthy adult life, well adapted to the environment. Yes, this can be very challenging. Yes, this can be frightening, but that is only because you have limited knowledge, and thus faith, in the unlimited potential for healing life and substance given to you by the energetic life force which created you. The intricate wisdom which runs each of the thousands of chemical reactions that go on in each one of your body cells, *each and every second of the day,* knows far better than any limited, educated, and ego/greed centered perspective on how to keep the body in a healthy, harmonious homeostasis with the Earth and environment in which you were spawn.

One key phrase you should always remember; one that will get you back on track and keep you focused no matter what the challenge in life, is this;

If I have faith in anything, anything can happen. The sky is the limit. If I have faith in nothing, nothing will ever happen. I am limited only by the boundaries of my own thought.

Do you expect to get ill? Then you will. Do you have some kind of psychological dependence for staying ill? Then you will never get well. When you learn to trust the inner power which runs the physical body, over time you develop an actual *kinesthetic experience* of this very inner power within you, caring for you and keeping your body in perfect order.

Symptoms of any kind are the body's method of purification, alerting you to make a change in lifestyle somehow. Hippocrates, the father of medicine, wrote;

"Diseases of any kind are crises of purification, of toxic elimination. Symptoms are the natural defenses of the body. We call them diseases, but in fact they are the cure of diseases."

Our family has observed first hand that allowing your children to go through illnesses and come out the other end produces an array of benefits, psychologically, physically and intellectually. They really do *grow* through the experience quite naturally, and we often notice greater, more advanced intellectual and physical shifts as a result.

"One of the best ways to ensure your children's health is to allow them to get sick. At first hearing this concept may sound outrageous. Yet, childhood illnesses, such as measles, mumps, and even whooping cough, may be of key benefit to a child's developing immune system, and it is inadvisable to suppress these illnesses with vaccines. Evidence is also accumulating that routine childhood vaccinations may directly contribute to the emergence of chronic problems such as eczema, ear infections, asthma, and bowel inflammations."

Philip Incao, MD medical researcher

"Contracting and overcoming childhood diseases are a part of a developmental process that actually helps develop a healthy, robust, adult

immune system able to meet the challenges that inevitable encounters
with viruses and bacteria will present later on."

Harris Coulter, Ph. D. from Vaccination,
Social Violence and Criminality. 1990

"There is no need to protect children from contracting infectious
diseases of childhood. These diseases are there to prime and mature their
immune system. Chronic ill-health, colds, otitis media, and upper and
lower respiratory tract diseases are well-documented in vaccinated
children. A well nourished child will go through rubella, whooping
cough, chicken pox and all the rest with flying colors."

V. Scheibner: Immunization:
The Medical Assault on the Immune System:
Australia 1993

"Vaccination subverts the immune system's natural response; the
ability to clear that virus. The rash is the body's eradication of the virus.
If you do not have a typical measles rash you are not invoking an
adequate cellular immune response. Measles may persist in the body
then. Children who do not develop the rash have an excess risk of delayed
mortality."

Andrew Wakefield, MD: NVIC Conference, 2002

Chapter Ten
Those pesky epidemics

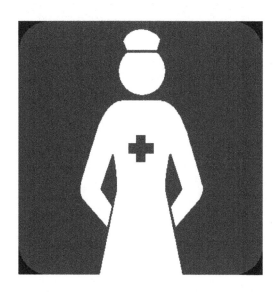

If germs don't cause disease, then why are there epidemics? We have already discussed briefly, the fraudulent production of epidemics for profit, engineered by the Epidemic Intelligence Service (EIS). Now, let's dive a little further into the nature of epidemics.

We have discussed that germs are ubiquitous, that you need them, and they are always fulfilling their function, which is to break down garbage that your body is attempting to eliminate.

If you still need some convincing after reading this far, consider this. If germs create disease, and indeed they are with us all the time, then why don't we always have some form of epidemic to deal with? What do medical professionals say about this? If you ask your medical doctor, she'll tell you there are certain factors that make germs more or less virulent at different times. Doesn't this mean then, that different germs require different factors in order to make them more or less virulent? If they do require these certain groups of circumstances to be virulent, aren't these factors the actual cause of disease, and not the germ itself? If not, then how come we have a pneumonia epidemic, and not a pertussis? Or measles epidemic, and not diphtheria?

Simply observe what happens when you are in whatever environment, and there is said to be "a cold going around." A lot of people can be ill, and one or two can be healthy. Or, one or two can be sick and the rest can be fine. What exactly determines this? Is it arbitrary? If indeed, everyone is getting sick at the same time, does this mean that they were all invaded by the same germ at approximately the same time? What made this germ decide to infect a bunch of people at the same time, and not others who may have been in the same place? Most medical professionals have never entertained such questions, because it is simply against their creed to think in such terms.

The popular argument that always comes up is, *individual resistance*. It is said that the reason all this occurs the way it does, is that some people are more resistant to infections, and thus epidemics, than others. I was more resistant than Sally, so she got sick and I didn't. But what exactly is *resistance*? Where does it come from? The immune system, like everyone talks about? If this is the answer, than aren't the factors that determine immune system resistance, or weaken it, the causative factors of disease, and not the germ?

If it is truly a matter of resistance, then why does one person get pneumonia, and another person gets measles? Is it a qualified resistance? If resistance is truly lowered, than why don't people get pneumonia, measles and diphtheria all at once? The reason, is because the germ theory is a load of krapp.

Since Bechamp's time and work, about 50 researchers world wide have worked on his idea of *pleomorphism* (many shapes for the same entity organism) and *spontaneous generation of micro-organisms through a more common body*, of which Bechamp called the Microzyma. This is in direct opposition to Pasteurian thought, which the medical cartel so vitally needs to hold on to if it is to stay alive and super wealthy. As you already know from the previous chapters, Pasteur insisted that micro-organisms were *monomorphic* (one shape only) and the sole causative factor in disease. There is a rumor that on his death bed, Pasteur denied all his previous theories and said that Bechamp was right. But then again, this is only a rumor.

Many researchers since the 1940's, in both the U.S. and Canada, have worked with Riffe's idea of UV radiation viewing scopes. They have all found things that you cannot see while using standardized culture and bacteriological viewing techniques with the common light microscope or electron microscope. These standardized techniques used in mainstream labs only view dead material. Using the full spectrum UV light and *dark field* scopes however, one can view the nature of blood and other tissues in their *alive,* natural state. Switching the focus from examining dead tissue, to examining living, makes all the difference in the world. If you are trying to help living people, doesn't it make sense to view living tissue samples? If you are trying to help people get and stay healthy, doesn't it make sense to study the body, tissue and cell in a state of *total health?*

Anyway, Bechamp's Microzyma have been found many times using these methods; one Canadian scientist, who continues his research to this day, also renamed them as *somatides.* These basic units of microbial life are found throughout living, healthy cells and tissues. When the body undergoes any level of stress, these small units seem to undergo a level of bacterial evolution to meet the needs of the individual. In our modern age of *science and research,* I call for a complete study of these basic units of life, and a total recount on the true nature of microbes.

We had mentioned before a very quiet branch of the CDC they call the *Epidemic Intelligence Service, or EIS,* which began in the late 1950's. These individuals are trained medical personnel, usually fresh out of school, that are sent to various State and local health agencies across the country. In these positions, they act as the eyes and ears for the CDC. Their job is to promote the party line, and to identify small clusters of disease incidence that can be turned into *"epidemics",* and further terrify the people into submission. From his book, *"Rethinking AIDS,"* Brian Ellison wrote:

"New graduates of medical schools and biological graduate schools are recruited upon graduation to take a several week course, and then dispatched on two year assignments paid for by the CDC. In various local and State health departments, they become an invisible intelligence network that watches for the tiniest clusters of disease, upon which are turned into national emergencies when the CDC deems appropriate. We saw this kind of manipulation in the 1957 Asian flu epidemic, and with clusters of leukemia in the 1960's which were attempted to appear as infectious by the CDC. We saw this occur with the swine flu "epidemic" that never materialized in

*1976, and with the legionaries "epidemic" that same year. We've
seen it more recently with lymes disease and viral pneumonia. After
the initial two years, every member of the EIS becomes part of a
permanent reserve officer core for the CDC, that can be called up
in time of war or national emergency, with actual emergency powers
under FEMA (the federal emergency management act . . . . a big
brother tool of confiscating everything everywhere during a declared
"national emergency"). Today, many of these people, by sitting in
foundations of major companies, the media, the Surgeon Generals
office, and other key positions politically act as advocates for the
CDC, echoing their view point whenever it needs support."*

I am old enough to remember when the CDC attempted to
declare leukemia as contagious in the mid 1960's. They actually
continued this effort, spending a lot of time and money on it,
through the later portions of the 1970's. But this effort backfired,
most likely due to the efforts of noble and honest researchers who
would not be bought. All they could muster up was a *"contagious"*
amongst cats form of leukemia called *feline leukemia syndrome.* If
they had been able, or ever are able to declare cancer as *"contagious,"*
the results will be devastating to public freedom. Once they
convince lawmakers that cancers can be contagious, they will come
up with a vaccine that no doubt will be made mandatory by law
for **all to receive,** in order to prevent a *"cancer epidemic."* Being it
known that the present vaccines used have already increased the
cancer rate astronomically to epidemic proportions, you can well
imagine how this new vaccine would further enhance the cancer
epidemic into pandemia. This is a very real scenario the medical
cartel may again decide to take up one day.

Anyway, getting back to the EIS, in 1992 because of too many
outside requests for the membership directory of the EIS, the CDC
has repressed availability of this directory. The CDC no longer
wants people knowing of the EIS membership, especially when we
have discovered that many of these people hold high media
positions. The head medical writer of the New York Times in 1994,
Larry Altman, was a graduate of the 1960's EIS. Every Surgeon
General is as well a graduate. Are you getting an idea of why you

do not read about the harmful effects of vaccines in the New York Times? Do you now have an idea of why the Surgeon General never makes a public statement regarding the dangers of vaccines? These people are groomed for influential positions for a very long time. They are an interesting form of *"career politician."*

The common denominator of problem with all the diseases we have discussed up to this point, is rooted firmly in the conception of the *germ theory*. Consider polio, aseptic meningitis, the flu, lymes disease, pneumonia, lupus and AIDS. What do all these diseases have in common? The answer is, they all have ***identical symptoms***. The only possible difference between them being their symptoms are switched around a bit in order, when referenced in any popular diagnostic text. Essentially, all these diseases are part of the same detoxification process, which renders them practically identical. In fact, when referenced in these texts, such as the *PDR* or the *Merck manual*, one has to logically wonder how on Earth a doctor is able to distinguish between these diseases. Diagnostically, and judgmental, they accomplish this task through their confirmatory antibody tests. Antibody tests ruin peoples' lives unnecessarily every day. They believe they have a possibly contagious, perhaps even socially awkward disease, and this single erroneous blood test has the power to throw any gullible life down the toilet. Or worse, as was the case with the popular tennis player *Arthur Ash*, kill you from the administration of a deadly "cure" for a disease that doesn't exist. By my rule book, Arthur Ash was murdered because he received erroneous information.

In the end, you must understand that the medical cartel is not really about applying treatment according to the guidelines of the germ theory, or any particular theory in general. They are about brain washing the public for profit, and they must maintain the germ theory in order to do this. This is not to say that all drugs are bad and all medical professionals are crooked. Nothing could be further from the truth. There are many cases in the honest practice of medicine where pharmaceutical intervention is vitally necessary, especially during times of crisis and emergency. In my 22 plus years of private practice, I have known most medical doctors to be very hard working and dedicated individuals. However, I believe that the bulk of medical practitioners are overworked, under paid (thanks to managed care), highly stressed and misguideded.

There is a wonderful allegory which explains the plight of medical professionals quite well. In this story, a man is walking along a rapidly flowing river, hoping to find a good fishing spot. Suddenly, he hears the panic of a man who is attempting to release himself from the rapids in the middle of the river. He looks further, and sees the man really needs help, otherwise he may well drown. So being a good swimmer, he jumps in to help the man. But it is nearly too late. When he reaches the man, he finds him unconscious. He quickly drags him back to shore, pumps the water out of his lungs and performs CPR. The man starts releasing the water and breathing again. He saved his life! But before the rescued man can come to his senses enough to thank the man who just saved his life, another scream is heard from the river. Now the rescuer sees two more people in the river, yelling for help. He again jumps in, and with more effort, saves them both. But just when he thinks it's all over, four more people are coming down the river, screaming for help. The man jumps in again, saving two and then reaching out a tall branch for the others to grab on to. They all made it to shore safely! What a hero! But then again, suddenly he hears the screams of 6 more people thrashing down the rapids and calling for help. You see, this hero is made so busy saving lives, that he doesn't have the time to walk up stream and find out who's throwing these people in.

The medical cartel is throwing them in, and laughing all the way to the bank. Should it be any wonder to you that *the majority of members of the FDA and CDC "oversight committees" have financial ties to vaccine manufacturers!* Some are found to even hold patents on vaccines presently under development. This is proof enough for *at least* a motive of why these highly toxic vaccines are pushed on children, despite overwhelming evidence which shows they should be taken off the market immediately. One person dies *supposedly* from a bad batch of the milk derivative *tryptophan*, which has been sold at health food stores for decades, and the FDA immediately jumps in and removes it from all shelves, in order to *"protect the public."* With thousands of adverse vaccine reactions being reported each year, ***the FDA does absolutely nothing*** to help save America's children. Both the FDA and CDC need to be closed down for their blatant misuse of power, and war crime trials similar to the Nuremberg trials of Nazi Germany after WWII need to begin against the many guilty members, responsible for maiming and killing thousands of children world wide.

Chapter Eleven

Got Research?

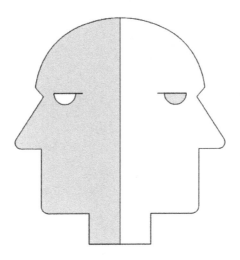

Got research!? How much does one need after all you've just read? Common sense being what it is, simply by virtue of the fact that vaccines contain one of the most toxic substances know to living cells, *MERCURY,* should tell you all you need to know. But of course it goes far beyond this. Many people will go through an adjustment period of denial, where they tell themselves over and over again that all this just can't be so. This is normal. Let yourself go through the doubt while you keep reading and investigating what you have learned here. It will pass. You may start thinking I am writing this book simply to get rich some how (what a laugh that is) by defaming the medical profession and pharmaceutical companies. Or maybe I have some deep personal grudge against the medical profession because I am a Chiropractor who just couldn't cut med school (a bigger laugh). Or maybe yet, I have way too much free time on my hands and nothing better to do. Well, when this finally passes you will then get very angry, especially since you trusted your medical provider who gave your children those very shots that have endangered their well being. Then you too will want to do something about it, and join the cause.

Well, if your nervous system hasn't been too damaged already by vaccines you probably have a good understanding that staying up late to finish and update this manuscript is no party. I am a family man with two absolutely beautiful un-vaccinated, un-medicated children to care for, and a beautiful wife of nearly 10 years who goes to bed on her own these nights I feel the obsessive pull to once again deliver this information to those who can benefit from it . . . . namely you! God asks me to do it (it is never a demand), so I do it. Given the time and capitol needed for printing and publishing, I just hope to break even (I have yet to check).

Believe me, I can think of a million things I would rather be doing right now. My kids are already fine. Yours are another question.

I travel around my small home town and see damaged children everywhere. Mind you, it takes a discerning eye to tell they have been dulled by vaccine poisoning at times; but it's there in mostly all the children I meet. Having two un-vaccinated, un-poisoned children gives me a perspective which makes these signs so obvious. There is a world of difference between vaccinated and non-vaccinated children in appearance, vibrancy, sharpness, alertness, and most obviously from the perspective of physical health. Un-vaccinated children get sick as they are supposed to by nature, and they get over their illnesses far quicker than vaccinated children, and develop a natural, lifetime immunity to illness and a strong immune system.

The artificial immunity purported by vaccine advocates is a total sham; it produces nothing but disease and couldn't even hold a candle to naturally developed immunity. I write this book; I travel and take further time away from my loving family life because I believe this is one of the most important issues of our time, and hardly anyone is speaking up about it. Seeing is believing, and my sole motivation is to show you the truth so your children can heal. I have seen how healthy my children are, and how unhealthy all the other vaccinated children are; and the gap grows wider each year. You need to get yourself and your children off all vaccines immediately, clean up their diets, give them a lot of good quality water and foods, and watch the magic happen. If they've had a bunch of vaccines they will most likely go through a detoxification period, but in most cases the body can bounce back in a short period of time (granted they haven't been too overly poisoned by vaccines already), especially if you consult the services of a local Naturopath, Chiropractor or other natural health practitioner to aid in the healing process. Oral *Proteolytic enzymes* can aid in the healing process in most cases. Check with your natural practitioner for dosages and indications.

Research is one of those very very very grey areas of life. If you think you're smart you always ask for the research. If you don't think you're smart you rely on someone else dictating it to you.

We make all our decisions based on some form of inquiry or *research* I suppose, even if it's as simple as your grandmother telling you I am the best Chiropractor in town and you should come and see me. You trust your grandma, she wouldn't lie to you, so you come and see me. You go past 20 Italian restaurants to get to this one across town that has the best marinara sauce you've ever tasted. But then one evening you are munching on your ziti and find a used band-aid. What do you do? Do you just forget about it, fling the used band-aid aside and continue to enjoy your meal? Do you ask the waitress to bring it back, give you a new entrée and simply try to forget about it? Or do you get totally grossed out, want to puke and never come back?

The point to all this is that it's totally up to you. There are so many variables to consider sometimes even with the simplest of decisions. At all times, you have to weigh out what's important; what really matters to you. Yeah, there was a gross used band-aid in your ziti marinara, but you've been eating there for 10 years and have never had a problem before. Or maybe the owner is a friend and you say nothing to keep the peace. Or maybe you're the kind of person that just can't tolerate anything like that even once. The point is, you take all the information and finally decide what is important to you. With concern to the main subject of this text, what can be more important than your health, or the health of your children? No matter how much you've been trained, or better said, brainwashed, to believe in the medical religion of the Illuminati, fact of the matter is that it is running you and your family into a deep, dark and deadly ditch that gets worse each year. Take the steps necessary to learn something new. Open your mind to the possibility that you have been lied to for many years about the nature of your body and your environment; that you are not the frail and fragile biological instrument that falls apart every time someone sneezes in your direction. Your body and immune system is a mastery of perfection, and the emperors are truly not wearing any clothes. It's time you too let them know you know.

This whole idea of "Research" is so ambiguous from the get go in any present human endeavor, that it's nothing but a joke, especially pharmaceutical research. Drug companies *expect* their researchers will find a favorable result for their products, if they want to keep their jobs and grants anyway. It is extremely rare that a drug company will ask a private research group to conduct testing on any of their products, and as far as I am aware this has never been done with vaccines. Private research groups have done many studies on vaccines, but the capitol for such endeavors has always come out of their own pockets. These are the groups that repeatedly tell us vaccinated kids are among the sickest in the world.

Ambiguity is a key word when contemplating research. Anyone can read or alter research data in any way to read anything they want if they are not properly checked and held to honest methods of data collection. Drug companies are rarely checked for research efficacy by the FDA. Oh they get an occasional slap on the wrist now and then for media window dressing (the very media they own), but for the most part the pharmaceutical industry is one of the most unchecked, un-audited, free to do what-ever-they-please industries that has ever existed, second only to the Internal Revenue "Service."

There's a very old joke about research scientists who were hired by the "Legs Don't Matter Company," to discover what would happen to a fly if it had all of it's legs surgically removed. Mr. Simon Swindel, CEO of the company, has been trying to convince people for years that his expensive walking machines, which do all the work for you, are far better than legs. Someone told him he needed more research on his side to better push his point, so he gave these researchers a big check from the LDM company, along with a strong hand shake and a wink. The head researcher winked back, and told Mr. Swindel to come back in one week.

So twelve researchers gathered around this poor little fly and began his demise. One researcher removed the first of his legs, and then yelled to the fly, "JUMP!" The fly did jump with very little difficulty. Everyone wrote down many notes. Then another researcher took off yet another leg, and yelled, "JUMP!" Somewhat more feebly but still okay, the fly again was able to jump. Everyone wrote down even more notes. Then a third researcher repeated the same procedure, removing one leg and yelling, "JUMP!" Again as before, the fly was able to jump. Well this went on until the poor fly had only one leg left, and surprisingly enough he was able to jump with it. Then another researcher removed the final leg, and yelled, "JUMP!"

The fly did nothing.

"JUMP!"

Still, he did nothing.

"JUMP!"

Still, he did nothing.

"JUMP I SAID DAMN YOU!"

Again, the fly did nothing.

Then all the researchers gathered together and yelled several dozen times as loud as they could.

"JUMP! JUMP! JUMP! JUMP! . . . . "

The result was the same, as the fly just lay there somberly.

So the researchers prepared an extensive report for the "Legs Don't Matter Company," and very excited about the results they called Mr. Swindel. With a big smile Mr. Swindel returned, this time with several associates. Smiling at the chief researcher, he asked, "so, what did you find?"

The researcher replied, "well, it was quite fascinating. We have discovered that the basis of existence for your LDM Company is quite valid, since our research shows that legs really don't matter. When you remove all of a fly's legs, he apparently goes stone deaf, since he no longer was able to hear our very loud commands. As a remedy for that, we researchers highly recommend that you expand your business into the sale of hearing aids with every walking machine."

It is my fervent belief that this is the true nature of all pharmaceutical research today. With that in mind, lets dive into some more important quotes and facts you will never hear on the evening news.

"Our children face the possibility of death or serious long term adverse effects from mandated vaccination programs that aren't necessary, or that have very limited benefits."

Jane Orient, MD
Executive director of the Association of
American Physicians and Surgeons

1997: New Zealand Journal of Medicine:

"Infant vaccination creates a high risk factor for allergy and asthma . . . ." This study found vaccinated populations of children to have 23% more asthma and 30% more allergies when compared to non-vaccinated children.

1994: Journal of the American Medical Association (hereinafter, JAMA)

This study showed that 11% of vaccinated children had asthma and developed pertussis, as compared to 0.8% of unvaccinated children.

2002: Thorax Medical Journal

This study showed that vaccinated children have 14 times more asthma and 10 times more eczema when compared to non-vaccinated children.

2000: Feingold MD, Research group

Demonstrated that 26% of vaccinated children have asthma as compared to 2% of non-vaccinated. 50% of vaccinated children had allergies as compared to less than 1% of non-vaccinated.

2001: Center for Science in the Public Interest

The vitamin K shot routinely given at birth is 50 times the normal *adult* dosage, besides being a synthetic chemical injected directly into a newborn's blood stream. Excess vitamin K is linked to liver cancer and leukemia.

2002: VAERS Report to federal government

244,424 reports of vaccine damage to children included the following;

99,145   emergency room visits
5,149   life threatening reactions
27,925   hospitalizations
5,775   disabilities
5,309   deaths

. . . . and this is just what was reported. If you want true national figures for these damage rates I would multiply each figure by at least 20. The above figures account for 59% of the total reports. The reported death rate in this sample was 2%.

Remember that under reporting vaccine damage is a huge problem in developing statistical truth. Death certificates do not record vaccines as the culprit of childhood demise and states under report vaccine related deaths by at least 100 times. If your child drops dead from a shot they received 20 minutes prior, the death certificate will state the child died of the disease he was vaccinated for, rather than the toxic shot he just received. According to a private Japanese study, under reporting of vaccine damage to children was discovered to be over 500 times in England.

1990: Harris Coulter, Ph.D. Center for Empirical Medicine
"15% to 20% of American school children are considered learning disabled with minimal brain damage directly caused by vaccines."

1998: JAMA
98% of children with pertussis were vaccinated for the disease in this study.

1989: Morbidity and Mortality Report
Discovered that pertussis outbreaks occurred in 100% vaccinated populations.

1986: Morbidity and Mortality Report
80% of measles outbreaks occurred in vaccinated populations

2000: Danish Study
"The increase in pertussis incidence is higher amongst vaccinated populations than it is in non-vaccinated populations of all ages."

1988: JAMA
"There is substantial under reporting of pertussis in the united states. Pertussis occurs at a far greater rate now than before the introduction of the vaccine."

1987: Journal of Epidemiology
Out of 137 cases of childhood measles studied, 99% were vaccinated for measles.

1999: British Medical Journal
Since the onset of Hib vaccination programs in England, incidence of infections has increased 4 fold. *"The potential risk of this vaccine far exceeds the potential benefits."*

Regarding Tetanus:
Incidence of this disease had declined by 92%, due to better hygiene and public sanitation, long before the vaccine was created between 1850 and 1900.

1990: New Zealand study
MMR vaccination programs this year created a tremendous outbreak of spinal meningitis.

2000: Journal of Epidemiology
Brazilian meningitis outbreak was discovered to be created by MMR vaccination programs.

1976: Ivan Illich, Ph. D., from the book Medical Nemesis. Chapter 1-Bantam Books
"Nearly 90% of the total decline in mortality for scarlet fever, diphtheria, whooping cough, and measles between 1860 and 1965

occurred before the introduction of antibiotics and widespread immunization."

To repeat a passage from chapter six:

With regards to all these old statistics used by the pharmaceutical companies in the 1950's and 1960's to "prove" vaccines wiped out the disease they were given for, the reader needs to understand as fundamental knowledge that all these early statistics from 1880 to 1965 showed a huge decline in disease incidence *NOT* due the administration of any vaccine, but due to advancements at this time in sanitation and public hygiene; i.e., less crowding of living spaces, better nutritional education, cleaner running water, plumbing for bath, shower and human waste. A generalized increase in the quality of living conditions occurred at this time in the history of western civilization, and these early, very dirty pharmaceutical companies jumped in to take credit for the health these things produced, stating it was due to their products that humanity was now saved from the scourge of these diseases. Every time the medical cartel quotes an example of how great vaccination programs are, they will do so using a statistic from 1910 to 1930, stating that thousands of children were dying of the said diseases at this time. Whereas this is true, looking at any graph from 1880 to 1970 will show that 1910/1930 disease rates were already on a steep decline from the earlier years as public hygiene and sanitation industry grew.

Vaccination programs for the mass public were not introduced until the mid 1950's in all cases you research; not until the tail end of the graph when the disease was decreased by over 90% from the beginning of the graph period (usually beginning at 1880 to 1900).

When considering the psychological profile of the parents and grandparents from that time period between 1950 and 1970; the one's whose children (like me) received the prototypical dosages of mass vaccination, you can understand how easy they were fool. Mostly all of them were traumatized from either the direct experience, memory or story of some family member maimed, paralyzed or killed from one of the dreaded diseases. Now here come these pharmaceutical representatives, fully understanding this psychological climate and taking full advantage of it's effects on local and federal government officials. Far less people had any of these diseases, but fear of them still reined free and true. Now here come the saviors! Those altruistic and hard working medical scientists, who will save society and quell your fears about these terrible things happening to you or your children. These early pharmaceutical representatives were nothing more than the progeny of snake oil salesman from the turn of the 20th century. You can just picture them there in the early days, standing on their soap boxes in the middle of the road; *"Just one shot my good friends will give you all the protection and peace of mind you need! You don't need to do anything else! We'll take care of you and your family from this point forward!"* Well, we all know how that "protection" truly worked out now, don't we. More disease instead of less, as those very diseases were already fully declined. More heartache and loss with the birth of a generation of neurologically and brain damaged children, directly caused by their "cures."

The standard M.O. for disguising their fraud throughout these early years of mass vaccination horror, a practice which occurs still to this day in the 21st century, was to train doctors and other medical cartel representatives *not to diagnose the said disease any more after the vaccination programs were administered, even if the exact same symptoms showed up in medical offices after the shots were administered. If it looked like polio after the polio shot was given, it just couldn't be polio anymore. It had to be something that a vaccine was not given for like spinal meningitis. If it looked like measles, it just couldn't be anymore. It had to be an allergic rash of some form or another. This practice alone of manually altering statistics and reporting is responsible for much of the public confusion centered around*

mass vaccination programs today, and the sole reason they are
still promoted as gospel.

2002: Neil Z. Miller, from his book "Vaccines-are they really safe
and effective?"

Before the onset of mass vaccination programs, measles was
already decreased by 98%, and pertussis by 99%. Scarlet fever,
typhoid fever and pertussis were once major killers, yet no vaccine
was produced for either scarlet fever or typhoid fever, and all three
scourges declined to virtually zero before vaccination programs were
promoted.

To repeat again from chapter 6:

Public officials always declare doom and gloom would be the
result it vaccination programs were to stop. But experience tells us
something different. Typically when pertussis vaccination is
decreased in different parts of the world, as was done in 1981 by
Sweden and the U.K., pertussis death rates actually dropped
dramatically in both countries, England reporting the lowest death
rates in recorded history. More whooping cough was diagnosed in
these areas during this period however, and this is another fine
example of how a promoted psychological climate from the medical
cartel alters reality, and creates a false sense of trouble favorable for
their products. When it was introduced that pertussis vaccination
programs would be decreased or eliminated as a test, medical and
pharmaceutical cartel representatives spread panic by insisting
doctors look for a probable whooping cough (same as pertussis)
outbreak. Due to this panic, now every case of bronchitis and flu
that enters into the doctors office suddenly becomes whooping
cough. Due to the subjective nature of data recording in these
instances, increases in any specific disease are virtually meaningless
since you can't be certain which problem you are actually talking
about. In most cases throughout the world, doctors will refuse to
diagnose a disease in which a person has been vaccinated for. This
political bias alone is enough to alter statistics persistently showing
a false, yet favorable result for vaccines.

1998: HU Baker & J. Husler: Febrile infectious childhood diseases in the history of cancer patients and matched controls: Medical Hypotheses

"This study investigates the hypothesis that febrile infectious childhood diseases (FICD's) are accociated with a lower cancer risk in adulthood . . . . The study consistently revealed a lower cancer risk for patients with a history of FICD."

1991: U Able, N Becker & R. Angerer: Common infections in the history of cancer patients and controls: Journal of Cancer Research and Clinical Oncology.

"The association between infectious diseases and cancer risk was investigated. Those with carcinomas of the stomach, colon, rectum, breast and ovary were interviewed. A history of common colds or gastroenteric influenza prior to the interview was found to be associated with a decreased cancer risk."

1999: B Schlehoper, M Blettner, S. Preston-Martin. Role of medical history in brain tumor development . . . . :Int. Journal of Cancer

"Subjects who reported a history of infectious diseases like colds and flus showed a 30% reduction in risk of brain tumors."

2003: RA Vilchez: American Journal of Medicine

"SV40 (monkey virus found in polio vaccines) is accociated significantly with brain tumors, bone cancers, malignant mesothelioma, and non-Hodgkins lymphoma."

2002: Thomas Jefferson (no kidding!) MD. The Telegraph

"Most MMR studies are meaningless, investigator claims are useless. There is some good research, but it is overwhelmed by the bad. The public has been let down because proper studies on vaccinations have not been done."

1999: Glen Dettman, MD medical researcher

"Smallpox would never had been the problem it was if the smallpox vaccine was not invented and promoted. In populations where there was no vaccine there was no smallpox."

I would like to conclude this chapter with a quote from a traumatized mother, taken from Barbara Fisher's book; DPT, a shot in the dark. At the beginning of the chapter I went over, however whimsically, the varying reasons why I am spending my valuable time writing this text. Primarily, I want to die knowing I did something with my lifetime to prevent on this confused and tormented Earth, situations like this. I am now finished with my 5th update of this text, and have waited till the last minute to place in this horrific letter, since it makes me physically ill and I can barely stand to listen to it.

"Death from vaccination is neither quick nor painless. I helplessly watched my daughter suffer an excruciatingly slow death as she screamed and arched her back in pain, while the vaccine assaulted her immature immune system. The poisons used as preservatives seeped through her tiny body, overwhelming her vital organs one by one until they collapsed . . . . my beautiful, innocent, infant daughter, death by lethal injection."

Christine C.'s daughter died
24 hours after receiving a DPT shot

Chapter Twelve
We're from the government, and we're here to help you!

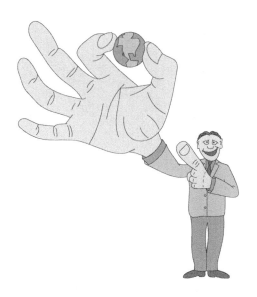

This chapter contains no legal advice. It does however, contain research for the purpose of education.

The founder of *Natural Hygiene* was a Naturopath named Dr. Herbert Shelton. He has many wonderful texts you can spend time learning with, and they are located in the reference section of this book. He said;

"The people shall be taught that they are free, and shall cherish the illusion all their lives. The greatest foe to the liberties of the people, is their own illusion of liberty."

Mostly everyone concerned about the vaccine dilemma comes face to face with their own personal battle with **BIG BROTHER**. I have written this book not only to give you the knowledge necessary to battle big brother bureaucracy, but to stand up for your God given and unalienable right to not be forcefully medicated, and to not have your children forcefully medicated against your will.

The Medical cartel has become a very powerful form of government that we all must stand up and speak out against. Using the political climate of 9-11, they now plan on moving their influence within government from one of "advisory power" to absolute power over decisions on what is best for you and your children; and or course, their toxic products reign supreme, as everything else more natural will be outlawed. They have many operatives in each state, that simply scare lawmakers into submission with erroneous data, with an end result being more deeply oppressive laws which force people to receive vaccines, and force parents to vaccinate children against their will. Putting it quite frankly, you have to become a bull dog with these issues if you wish to keep yourself, and your family free from harm. Until the day comes where they admit, "Okay, the nation is essentially bankrupt, you have no rights and will do whatever the state tells you to do, since it's for the good of the people," no one can legally force you, or your children, to be medicated against your will. No one! If we are truly a "free" society, you are not the pet of the state and will decide for yourself what is best for your family's bodies, so long as you don't disturb the health of anyone else. Some more aggressive medical cartel states, like New York, Maryland, Massachusetts and West Virginia, may insist you comply with standardized vaccine codes, but you always have a way out of their traps if you work at it hard enough. You will find examples of this in the remedies section of the book, which follows. For now, I will give you vital background information on how to fight and beat this oppressive vaccine system.

It sure seems at times, that many lawmakers are on the "payroll" of the medical cartel (by owning stock in companies, granted a position on a company board, receiving a huge grant by a company for supporting vaccine programs, not to forget a myriad of illegal "gift" transfers . . . . the list of rewards is endless for those who play the game). Over zealous ones, such as the now Senator (dear God!) Hillary of NY, are attempting to legislate vaccine program mandates on the federal level. If not done directly, they will attempt to slip these in under other legislation, right under the nose of the people, so be very careful to watch the particular politics of your state. As it is, they have most schools, and now colleges requiring vaccines for admission. They want to include a vaccine record of every person in America, if not the world, on a standardized data base to make sure they miss no one. This was the national health care card Hillary Clinton attempted to push on the American public through her national health care plan. The Medical cartel wants to refuse you airline travel, hotel and car reservation privileges if you refuse to receive your yearly dose of vaccines. They want us all to be their pets, caring for us by making sure we all have our shots. These are some very important issues to watch keenly in the years which follow this new century. Mark my word, if people do not stand up and speak out against such oppression and tyranny, it will happen sooner than you may think. Everyone will have a nice little vaccine giver show up at their door one day and say, "Hello, I'm from the government department of vaccinations, and I'm here to help you comply with the law today by getting you and your family up to date with your yearly vaccines. Would you like to sit or bend over?"

I have heard many horror stories over the years of practicing in the north eastern United States, that schools hassle parents who even question the validity of vaccines for their children. Several school officials even told parents in my practice that they would contact the DCF if they even dared do such an injustice to their children by not vaccinating them. Parents who refuse vaccinations for newborns at hospitals have also been reported to the DCF. Don't let this worry or intimidate you. You still have rights to exercise in this country regarding the issue, and no overzealous school nurse, principal or DCF flunkie can take those rights away. You will need to learn how to show your teeth however.

Understand right now, that our country was founded on creator endowed, unalienable rights that do not come from the constitution, but from God and nature. When the tax protesters, our early founding fathers, revolted to form our great nation, after the war was won they ended up attempting to discover a remedy on paper to make sure the tyranny they experienced would never happen again. This remedy was not the constitution of these united states, but the *federalist papers.* Any one of the founding fathers of the constitution could walk into congress today, and make them all look like the corrupted band of idiots they have truly become. The founding fathers were a collective of brilliant minds who knew what oppression and tyranny were. They knew they needed some form of centralized government to deal with issues like commerce between states and war, but that was it! They left the rest up to the individual states. When the treaty of peace was signed with Great Britain after the revolt, the document acknowledged that we were each given sovereign power, equal to the King individually. We in

America became sovereigns without subjects. Each man and woman
a sovereign in their own right, bowing only to God. Then came
the constitution, but the constitution does not give you any creator
endowed and unalienable rights. Only God can give you those.
This is the basis of what is called *the common law*. Your God given,
unalienable rights are exercisable under the common law, which is
the source of this country. The common law is based on the Bible,
both old and new testaments, primarily centered around the ten
commandments.

But where have we gone since this time? We used to be citizens
of our sovereign state, not federal citizens. The truth is, you are
still a citizen of your sovereign state. The constitution still defines
a very limited power to a centralized federal government, and we
were conceived and created as a **REPUBLIC**, not a democracy. In a
republic, you are a sovereign without subjects. In a democracy,
everyone votes to see what the majority wants, and elected officials
have more power over decisions that effect everyone's lives. There
is a big difference between the two. In truth, our constitution
provides that each state has powers far beyond those of the federal
government. But then our elected officials at the federal end got
involved with a bunch of international bankers, and we had a civil
war. We started borrowing money from European banks and getting
into immense debt. After the civil war came the 14th amendment,
which history claims is what freed the slaves from the south. Article
4, section 2 of the constitution reads;

*"The Citizens of each state shall be entitled to all privileges and
immunities of Citizens in the federal states . . . ."*

The 14th amendment reads;
*"All persons born or naturalized in the United States and subject
to the jurisdiction thereof, are citizens of the United States and of
the state wherein they reside."*

These 14th amendment citizens are spelled with a small "c."
The ones in the original constitution, Article 4 section 2, are spelled

with a capitol "C." Did you know there was a difference? A CAPITOL "C" **Citizen** is a state citizen with full common law rights. A 14th amendment, small "c" **citizen** is a federal citizen. If you consider yourself a 14th amendment small "c" citizen, then you are first and foremost a federal citizen, and not a sovereign. What does this mean? Well, the federal government *is* the United States. But there are three distinctly different United States as defined by the US supreme court. The first is the United States of America, which is the American *territory*. The second is the union of the several States, usually referred to as *"these united states,"* with the united states in all small letters, representing more of a location than an actual noun. The third is an artificial corporate entity, called the United States(or UNITED STATES), listed just as you see in beginning capitol letters or all caps. This is what is referred to as the federal government. They are actually a corporation which has been created for dealing with the details of doing business amongst the several states, and foreign policies such as war and the military. You will notice that 14th amendment citizens who have been naturalized, have all their rights granted to them by the constitution. But capitol "C" Citizens of the constitution had all their common law rights to begin with, and are *sovereigns in their own right first,* above and beyond any state or federal mandate. In a sense, 14th amendment citizens are more *federal* citizens, controlled by the laws formed by the federal United States corporation. Capitol "C" original Citizens are governed only by common law, the *original* constitution of these united states with the bill of rights, and the laws of their particular state. Don't think these small and capitol "C's" don't matter. This was carefully planned. 14th amendment citizens are subjects first of the federal government, and secondly to God, the common law, and the *FEDERAL* STATE.

Now, what does all this have to do with vaccines and your rights to not vaccinate? *We are all capitol "C" citizens, governed by the common law, unless we sign a contract in which we agree to trade those common law rights for some federally provided privileges.* This occurs every time you sign a 1040 tax form or the like, obtain a marriage license, and apply for a driver's license. You are always signing your common law rights away without even realizing you are doing so. No matter what anyone tells you, if you have to sign for something, that something is not mandatory. You are volunteering to participate in it. When you sign a marriage license, for example, your marriage is now a three way legal partnership between the man, wife and state. This is how the state steps in and "helps" you make decisions on vaccinating your children, because if you have a state marriage license, your children are one third the ward of the state. If you say no vaccines for my kids, and some over zealous medical doctor feels your decision to not vaccinate is child abuse, the state DCF can send police to your home, grab your kids and forcefully vaccinate them. There have been several cases in America, where the parents have refused medical care (none with vaccines as yet) for sick children with cancer, and the DCF stepped in, took the child and gave them the treatment against the parents will. Unless we are all very careful, soon they will be doing this with vaccines, and not only with children, but with adults as well. Children are a gift from God under the common law, and certainly cannot be taken from the parent because they refuse to medicate the way the state mandates. When you begin to assert your rights as a free, sovereign human being (as apposed to the all CAPITOL LETTERS SPELT "individual" or "person" which are corporate terms in commerce), you will realize how you are not a subject to any CODE LAW of the UNITED STATES corporation unless you intentionally contract with them.

WHO EXACTLY ARE YOU?

These points of *commerce and contract*, fall under a system of commercial law which some law researchers say has become the real "law of the land," called the Uniform Commercial Code, or UCC. The concepts centered around learning the UCC to protect yourself and your family are not difficult, but they are somewhat time consuming in the beginning, primarily due to the fact that most people need a sufficient amount of time to become at least moderately *unbrainwashed,* for lack of a better term. The average person has no concept of freedom such as the liberty outlined in the original constitution of these united states. He has a very difficult time comprehending that he can be a sovereign; a totally free human being living under the common law, if he so chooses and takes the appropriate steps to do so. First and foremost, you need to figure out who, on this Earth, you *truly* are.

Are you **JOHN QUINCY PUBLIC**, or **John Quincy Public**? Are you both? Did you know there was a difference? Have you ever noticed that the all capitol version of your given name appears on virtually every piece of "official" printing out there? Well, there is a HUGE difference between these representations of your being. The natural English language, upper and lower case version represents the living, breathing, flesh-and-blood being that you truly are. The one God created. The other all CAPS version represents a corporate trust entity, what is called a person or individual within commerce and corporate structure. This is who all governments would like you to believe you are.

The most fundamental principle to understanding the UCC, is that the powers that be already consider you a sovereign, but they keep it secret. They really don't want you knowing about it. They want to keep you in the dark about your freedom for, well, your entire life if they can, keeping you as a volunteer federal slave. It all begins at your birth, when your parents file a birth certificate with the state. That piece of paper is your entryway into federal serfdom, if you do nothing else to reclaim it.

From that birth certificate, the federal government, who illegally gave away congress's sole authority to coin gold and silver as real money, sets up a corporate trust account using the name you were given **IN ALL CAPITOL LETTERS** as a trust entity, and your labor as its value, as calculated by the money you will generate hypothetically throughout your anticipated lifetime. They then set up a *bond,* a trust instrument which states the value of a "thing" (namely, you), affix a value of currency to it, then offering it as collateral to the Federal Reserve Banking System. They use your birth certificate as a marker of labor, and then offer it as collateral to a privately owned corporation? Yes, that's exactly right. This is a softer definition of serfdom and slavery, but slavery nonetheless. Haven't you ever wondered why all official documents and licenses have a form of your name seen in all CAPITOL letters? This is not proper English, yet it is persistently done. Do you suppose it is a mistake, or just for no good reason? It is for a very good reason in fact. That ALL CAPITOL NAME is not you, the living, breathing flesh and blood human being. It is technically called your *straw man,* or the trust entity set up upon the filing of your birth certificate. This ALL CAPTIOL CORPORATE PERSON is who the powers that be what you to believe you are. You are not that "person" or "individual"; you are a naturally born human being with creator endowed common law rights, but you have to know this. If you do not, you default to their brand of corporate person slavery.

How can they do this? It all started in the late 1800's, when wealthy European bankers, members of the Illuminati of course, began sabotaging the gold and silver money flow in America. They again used the Hegelian philosophy, creating a problem, instituting and witnessing the reaction (fear and frustration), and then generously offering a solution. Their manipulation of the gold and silver markets led to several shortages which created havoc in the states. They offered a solution then, of their vast experience and expertise in the field of banking, suggesting they take control of the flow of currency in America through a centralized UNITED STATES corporate banking system. In this system, the bankers own the fiat (fictitious) money, which inherently has no value, especially when compared to gold and silver coin. Congress stops issuing gold and silver coin, and suspends their control of America's money supply indefinitely. Now, a privately owned corporation that is not part of the government will have the ability to own and control the flow of paper currency, lending it to the government for distribution amongst the people. The government can have as much as they want, but they will actually have to *borrow it* from the Federal Reserve Banks, with interest attached.

Sound like a deal you would take if you were a leader? No, I didn't think so. But the federal government finally caved in 1913, signing into effect the Federal Reserve Act, culminated with going off the gold standard illegally in 1933. Now the government had Federal Reserve Notes, or FRN's. These had to be paid back to the Federal Reserve Banks at a decided interest rate, and until the mid 1920's, that interest was to be paid in gold. What a great deal! They issue paper and get gold in return! Can anyone here say, robbery?

For years then, these European bankers were paid their interest sums in gold, shipped over from our resources on a regular basis. Then the mines ran low and the gold began to run scarce around the mid 1920's, and we could no longer pay the interest in this way. This was the primary cause of the *great depression*, which began in 1929. We couldn't pay the interest, so the European bankers stopped lending us their fiat, worthless paper money.

So to remedy this for the bankers in 1933, Roosevelt declared a national emergency and signed an executive order, which said every "person" and corporation needs to send in their gold to the federal government, to be exchanged for worthless paper script (FRN's). Of course, people did not know that they are considered *human beings, natural flesh and blood existing beings, and they were NOT PERSONS*. The word, *person or individual,* may include a natural, existing flesh and blood human being; but it could also simply mean any or all corporations. Of course, the executive order was not specific to this point. If in 1933, people knew to simply call the government on this point, they would have been able to keep their gold.

But that wasn't the case. People turned in their gold for worthless paper. The federal government then paid what they could to the bankers in gold to ease the debt, and offered an alternative plan for interest payment; *YOUR LABOR.* This was accomplished through a House Joint Resolution in 1933, called HJR 192. Within the tenets of this resolution, the legal gold and silver standard was to be suspended indefinitely; a completely illegal act since this portion of the constitution, rendering congress the full power of money creation, cannot be amended or suspended in any way. So these acts illegally became *public policy* (a very gray area of law), and paper money would now be the main currency of the UNITED STATES corporation, along with a myriad of other banking instruments such as bonds, promissory notes, drafts and bills of exchange. Only FRN's however, were the property of the bankers, loaned to the federal government at interest. The other debt elimination instruments could be made by anyone, not necessarily to *pay* for anything, but to discharge debts. You are able to create *credit*, and the federal government promises to discharge that credit with this fiat money.

The creators of HJR 192 were aware that trading your labor; i.e., using the hard earned wages of Americans as collateral and a substitute for the interest payment owed by the federal government, is simply another form of slavery. Isn't slavery supposed to be illegal in America? Well, yes it is. So they formulated a plan through HJR 192, which is not spelled out specifically this way but certainly implied, whereas all Americans would now have their debts totally paid off by the federal government since there was no longer *any legal money in existence*. You can go out and buy a TV with their worthless script (FRN's), and they will ensure payment for the item at some later date when the gold standard returns. That is the entire concept behind FRN's. They pay NOTHING! How can they? They are not backed by anything with intrinsic value, like gold, silver, or even simple rocks! They are essentially, *instruments of debt owed by the federal government to the bankers.* They are only backed by your supposed labor power over your lifetime, and the promise that the government will pay for the debts they incur at some later date. Sound confusing? Well, it is! It was meant to be this way.

So Federal Reserve Notes are paper you can now use for legal tender, for the payment of public and private debts. You go buy stuff with them when you are able to work for enough of them, and by handing them to someone you are essentially saying, "the government told me they will pay me when the gold standard comes back, so when that happens I will pay you as well." Then that person hands the paper you just gave him to someone else, and he to someone else, and the cycle goes on and on. Over the decades, people have totally lost sight of how this system should be working, but back in the early days, plenty of people knew and were not very happy about it. This is why HJR 192 needed to provide an *exemption, or remedy* for the Americans who were now earning nothing of worth for their labor. The government says here, that the debts of Americans will be paid, dollar for dollar, in whatever currency the government says is legal tender. It was now against public policy for anyone to ask for any **specific** form of payment.

Your remedy is exactly this, offered by HJR 192 of 1933. If you incur a debt from a credit card, loan, or a credit account at the local store, that debt can be discharged with any number of debt elimination instruments made legal by the federal government's banking laws. You can choose to pay with FRN's, but don't have to if you choose to use another legal instrument. Well, if you choose to pay with a bond, or bill of exchange of some legal form, what is backing that up? This is where your birth certificate comes into the game. It was "sold," in a matter of speaking, or used as collateral, for the debt owed to the bankers by the federal government. Joe Blow is born, and his parents file a birth certificate. That certificate is a receipt of property, now filed with the **department of commerce, and used as a receipt of collateral for the bankers.** The **JOE BLOW** *"corporate person" (a business trust created by the feds),* will most likely make 1.5 million dollars in his lifetime, and this amount will be depreciated by ongoing (illegal) taxation, and paid directly to the Federal Reserve Banking system to pay off the interest incurred by the federal government for using FRN's. This is how it all works, and exactly why the so called *national debt* will never go down until we return to the gold standard, and stop giving this ridiculous level of power to the Federal Reserve Banking system.

For more direct information and discussion on the banking system, and how to become free in your business and personal affairs, research the following information:

Phone DESM @ 954-934-0304

Other related web sites are;

www.lawresearchgroup.com
www.zerodebts.com
www.freeenterprisesociety.com
http://beam.to/tapes (note there is no www. on this one).
These folks are affiliated with the Republic of Texas, and can also be reached at;
Tapes/Info
c/o P. O. Box 412
Princeton, Texas [75407]
972-504-8705
texanlae@yahoo.com

Obtain all the study materials which pertain to you. This out of print book called, "Cracking the Code," 3rd edition, will also be very useful if you can find it on a google search. Specifically to accomplish freedom under the UCC, you need to know how to file the following documents as a part of public record (the people at DESM above are excellent at helping you with this process);

**COMMON LAW COPYRIGHT OF THE ALL CAPS
   TRUST NAME
POWER OF ATTORNEY FOR THE ALL CAPS NAME
NOTICE OF COMPETENCY FOR THE NATURAL
   HUMAN BEING
DECLARATION OF PERSONAL INDEPENDENCE
ACCEPTANCE OF THE OATH OF OFFICE OF ALL
   PUBLIC OFFICIALS**

The instructions for these filings can be obtained through the noted UCC study groups, and DESM.

The Uniform Commercial Code was built up around the concepts of HJR 192, and has become the supreme law of the land for commercial ventures; which for all intents and purposes accounts for everything. For the ALL CAPS individual or person (trust), even criminal charges like murder are commercial crimes. All laws today are in commerce, with the UCC reigning as supreme. But what about the united states constitution? Well, it reigns as the supreme law of the land as well, but you need to understand how, and claim the rights under it hereto. That constitution only applies to the natural born human being represented by the upper and lower case name. Unknowingly, you have volunteered to be known as the ALL CAPS trust corporate entity, and in so doing have waived all your constitutional rights, thus defaulting to make the UCC your supreme law of the land. Want to change that? Then begin studying the UCC with the given contacts, and get busy in the filing of your necessary paperwork.

How the supreme law of the land should work

Article 6, paragraph2 of the united states constitution is known as the SUPREMACY CLAUSE. It states:

"This constitution and the laws of the united states, which shall be made in pursuance thereof, and the treaties made or which shall be made under the authority of the united states shall be the supreme law of the land, and that judges in every state shall be bound thereby; ANYTHING IN THE CONSTITUTION OR LAWS OF ANY STATE TO THE CONTRARY ARE NOTWITHSTANDING (this means notwithstanding in law, or contrary to law).

The translation in modern times? First and foremost it means that the united states constitution is an iron clad contract between a limited, centralized federal government (the way it was designed to be), and the people. The people are the clear beneficiaries of this contract, and at all times you need to ask for the enforcement of this contract in your favor. Here is something strong to back you up:

Marbury vs. Madison: Key case @ 5 US 137:

Recorded at vol. 5 (1803) pg. 137, the judge in this case, John Marshall, chief justice of the supreme court, states that *anything which is in conflict with the constitution is null and void at law.* Does this include amendments made to the constitution by the congress? Yes it most certainly does. Does it include totalitarian acts, such as Patriots I & II, as well as all the preceding "anti-terrorist" acts? Absolutely. Clearly, this case sets a precedent which protects your original common law rights as declared by the original united states constitution. *"For a secondary "law" to come into conflict with the supreme law is totally illogical, for certainly the supreme law would prevail over all other law, and certainly our forefathers had intended that the supreme law would be the basis of all law, and for any law to come into conflict with the supreme law is null and void at law.* **It would bear no power to enforce, it would bear no obligation to obey, it would report to settle as if it never existed, for unconstitutionality would date from the enactment of such a law, not from the date so granted in a open court of law. No courts are bound to uphold it, no citizens are bound to obey it. It operates as a mere nullity of fiction, which means it does not exist in law."**

WOW! Pretty powerful and directly to the point, wouldn't you say?! How many "Acts, Bills, Titles, Codes," or any other kinds of "laws" can you think of that are in direct opposition of the original constitution today? It is supposed to be the supreme law of the land even today. Any oppressive vaccination bill which violates your right to privacy, and unwarranted search and seizure is also against the supreme law of the land.

SHEPARDS CITATIONS are a set of court recordings which keep track of all the court cases that have come and gone, especially within the supreme court. They clarify all of the cases that ever go before the courts. Marbury vs. Madison is standing very strong from its inception in 1803, over 200 years later in 2004. It has been used over 200 times, accounting for over 9 pages of this set of citations, and has yet to be overturned by any other case or judge.

As an American, you can only give up your constitutional rights by signing them away, which is what you have done time and time again without knowing. You need to learn where you are doing this and stop doing it. First and foremost is to not sign any form of license with the state for a marriage. Why would you want to do this? It alerts the government of your private information; volunteers you and your new spouse to give up your constitutional rights together and live by the laws of the UNTIED STATES corporation, and by the corporate charter of your particular state. When you sign a marriage license, the state is now a third party legally in your marriage. Your children, considered in common law as the property of the parents until adulthood, are now one third ward of the state. You have to consider them when making all decisions about your children's lives. If you make a decision which is contrary to what the state believes, they have a legal right to protect a piece of their property, your child, and step in whether you like it or not. If you truly want to protect your children and family from state vaccination oppression, the first thing you must do is rescind your marriage license through public declaration. Your marriage can be recorded in a Bible, or any other spiritual text of your choosing for posterity, which makes the union real in the eyes of God, and keeps the state out or your bedroom.

The supreme court has ruled in hundreds of cases that "the rights of the people" means the right of each and every human being equally. This has been especially true when defending the second amendment for bearing arms. The constitution says this right shall not be infringed, and there are no subparagraphs describing the ways of this infringement. Thus, it means ALL infringement shall be forbidden.

If someone ever tries to forcefully vaccinate you or your child, no matter what prima facae law (colorful law) may be pushed in your face, you must start yelling, and loudly;

1. I claim you are stealing my rights!
2. I claim infringement on my rights to life, liberty and happiness under the first amendment!
3. I claim impingement!
4. I claim encroachment!
5. I claim usurpation of my legal constitutional rights!
6. If you violate any of my constitutional rights I will sue and attach everything you own!

Dealing with the bad guys

Here are some more bureaucrat eliminators that have worked like Raid on roaches for people attempting to protect themselves from government, or any other "official" fraud, over the past few decades. They are great to use in tight situations;

1. "I want you to know that I fully accept your *Oath of Office* in this matter, and as a result I expect you to uphold all my unalienable rights."
2. "What gives you the authority to speak to me in this abusive manner?"(Or for that matter, what gives them the authority to speak to you at all?! Remember that any manner in which they speak to you is abusive if they do not have the proper delegated authority, and thus you are being damaged with every word)
3. "Where does your delegated authority come from to demand or ask these things of me? I would like to see that delegated authority immediately if we are to continue talking." (Be careful here, since they may simply flash a badge and say, "here is my authority." A badge means nothing. You have the right to see the delegated authority in writing before you speak to anyone demanding anything of you)
4. "Are you going to uphold all of my unalienable rights during the course of my interactions with you?"
5. "Alright, I claim that I am not resisting or evading my responsibilities in any way here. I accept your Oath of Office

in this matter, as well as what you are saying to me. *Kindly verify, in writing and signed under the penalty of perjury*, that you have the proper delegated authority to compel me to do everything you are asking me to do against my will, and I will comply." (To this day in Gregorian calendar history, no one has ever received anything from any "official" signed under the penalty of perjury. Another maxim under the common law is, *equality under the law is paramount.* If they are asking you to sign things under the penalty of perjury, you have the unalienable right, as well, to compel them to do the same. P.S., they will **NEVER** do this as long as the sun keeps rising in the sky, because 99% of all "officials" you meet act outside the boundaries of their delegated authority, assuming they even have any authority or an Oath of Office to uphold your rights and the constitution)

You need to understand who you truly are. You are a sovereign, free spiritual being that can not be pushed around by any bureaucratic thug, *but only if you claim that you are indeed, sovereign and free.* There is an old saying amongst freedom circles which applies to every day of your life;

If you don't know your rights, then you don't have any.

This is not whim, rather, it is an actual maxim of legal precedent. All your life, you have been trained by the corporate media to *"respect authority,"* to cooperate, and to go along to get along without asking any questions. This is how the average person lives as a slave; an **ALL CAPS** piece of trust property pledged to the money powers in this corporate matrix they call "life." Until you stand up and declare your freedom, you are indeed, a slave. Unless you say otherwise, you are indeed their **ALL CAPS** piece of property, void of any rights, and granted certain *privileges* upon good behavior as their slave.

You should **NEVER** answer any questions of anyone who claims authority over you. Here is the way this game is played;

> *He who asks the questions, and continues to ask the questions, wins.*

You should **NEVER** communicate about anything over the telephone. **ALWAYS** instruct the person on the other end of the phone that you do not do business in this way. Instruct them to place everything in writing and send it to you. When you receive their mish-mosh, write the following across it, returning the item(s) to them within 3 business days;

ACCEPTED FOR VALUE AS TRUE. I AM RETURNING THIS TO YOU FOR SETTLEMENT AND CLOSURE OF THIS MATTER FOR FAILURE TO STATE A CLAIM UPON WHICH RELIEF CAN BE GRANTED. I ACCEPT YOUR OATH OF OFFICE, AND I DO NOT WISH TO CONTRACT WITH YOU. IF YOU THINK YOU ARE REPRESENTING ME, YOU ARE HEREBY FIRED.

As an sovereign American, you can as well, claim your rights under Marbury vs. Madison as legal and true. The case has never been overturned after 201 years standing strong. You claim your rights from the constitution as you say they are, not as they say they are.

A strategy for dealing with school/DCF officials, including school lawyers, that are blocking your child's access to school

1. Get the exact names of the people blocking your child access to school.
2. Send a PUBLIC RECORDS ACT request to them on their authority to act as they do (see forms section)

3. Charge them $1000 if they do not answer request, and then $1000 per day for your damages and inconvenience if your child is still not allowed to attend school.
4. Invoice them for the amount owed to you after 30 days.
5. Follow up on the invoices as would a debt collector. For help on this procedure contact DESM @ 954-934-0304.

If you feel like you just cannot stand all this confrontation, here is something else you might try. It does not add to the greater good as far as educating people of this vaccine fraud running rampant, but at least you may be able to get your needs met.

If you are partial to using medical doctors instead of natural practitioners, and have developed a good relationship with some pediatrician, office nurse or physician assistant, you may try to simply educate him, in private, to the dangers of vaccines and thus your needs. I have noticed that in 50% of the cases this works well. A strategy I have often recommended, is the *"Orange Diversion."*

Work it out with whomever you have to in the office rendering the shots. Use your best communication skills and try not to be intimidating, demanding or authoritative. Do not waste your time talking to people who are ultra-brainwashed and thus unable to understand you. Sometimes you can bypass the busy doctors running around, because they let the nurses or physician assistants administer the vaccines. Obviously you only care about developing a relationship with the person giving the shots. In many cases you can get them to understand, even if they do not fully agree, that certainly if you do not want to have you children vaccinated you should not be forced to do so. Work all the details of the Orange Diversion out beforehand, and proceed simply as follows:

1. Bring your child(ren) in for their scheduled shots. Have a large orange or two in your purse or pocket.
2. Proceed as usual without attracting any attention to the situation. Just tell your kids they are going into the office for a check up and to otherwise shut up!

3. The doctor or nurse then gets the shots ready, records the lot numbers and everything else they do in your file, and brings the shots to your room as usual.

4. Keep the door closed, and be sure there are no security cameras spying on you. Then take out the oranges and inject them instead of your kids. Be sure to take the oranges with you (very important)! You walk out and everyone is happy. Be sure your kids keep quiet as you walk out and pay. The last thing you need is for innocent little Johnny to blurt out, "wasn't that funny how we gave the shot to the orange!"

The first amendment of the constitution talks about the pursuit of life, liberty and happiness. Doesn't the protection of your body, the maintenance of your body and the bodies of your children as you see fit fall under this right? You are not hurting anyone by refusing medical vaccinations, since it can not be proven that you, or your children are a hazard to anyone if you do not receive medical vaccinations, and you are able to prove this fact with an endless array of scientific fact. Here is another bureaucrat eliminator;

"Sir (Madam), what is it you do not understand about your Oath of Office to uphold and protect the constitution? You are aiding and rendering comfort to the enemy by breaking down the laws of our land and breaking your oath of office."

After all, according to Title 18 USC, section 2381, in the presence of two or more witnesses to the same overt act or in an open court of law, if you fail to timely move to protect and defend the constitution of these united states, and **honor your Oath of Office, you are subject to the charge of capitol felony treason.** As well, if any part of any bill or law are found to be unconstitutional, then the entire corpus of the bill is unconstitutional. Is there someone you assume has authority over you, using unconstitutional colorful "law" as a weapon against your liberty? Is there some phony "pseudo," or "colorful" official, stepping out of the confines of their Oath of Office to make your life a living hell? Why are you letting him or her ruin your life?

Your right to due process is found equally under the forth, fifth and sixth amendments. The forth states the right of people to be secure in their homes, specifically;

"The right of the people to be secure in their PERSONS, houses, paper and effects against unreasonable searches and seizures . . . . SHALL NOT BE VIOLATED . . . . and no warrants shall issue, but upon probable cause, supported by Oath or affirmation and the particularly describing the place to be searched and the persons or things to be seized."

From the ninth amendment:

"The enumeration in this constitution of certain rights shall not be construed to deny or disparage others retained by the people."

That is to say, your common law rights can not be violated in any way, shape or form without probable cause of committing some crime against the common law, by some measurable loss to some other living human being. **What this means is that congress has no authority whatsoever to add onto the constitution in such a way that would take any rights away previously guaranteed to anyone. If they do, according to Marbury vs. Madison, those very add on's, in whatever form they may be, are to be:**

1. Declared null and void
2. Recognized as having no power to enforce
3. Recognized as having no obligation to obey
4. Reported to settle as if they never existed
5. Known as unconstitutional from the date of enactment
6. Recognized as no court being bound to uphold them

The tenth amendment states;

"The powers not delegated to the united states by the constitution, nor prohibited by it to the states are reserved to the states respectively or to the people."

This means the constitution is a limited contract, meant to limit government. Nor do the police have the power to take away rights previously guaranteed by the constitution. **Marshall vs. Kansas City Mo., 355 S.W. 2nd, 877,883** states;

> *"Police power is subject to limitations of the federal and state constitutions, and especially to the requirement of due process."*

Some other great facts to remember are;

Title 5, USC section 556 (d): also 557, and section 706: If you are denied due process of law in any way, all jurisdiction ceases automatically.

From American Jurisprudence, volumes 16: Constitutional Law, section 97:

This volume tells a judge how to interpret the constitution;

> *"That the constitution should receive a liberal interpretation in favor of the citizen is especially true with respect to those provisions which were designed to safeguard the liberty and security of the citizen in regard to both PERSON and property . . . ." See note 31, Breyers vs. United States 273 US 28 . . . . "and a constitutional provision intended to confer a benefit should be liberally construed in favor of the clearly intended and expressly designated beneficiary (you!). Similarly a provision intended to afford a remedy to those who have just claimed should receive a beneficial construction for the purpose of extending the remedy to all who might fairly come within the meaning of the terms."*

Forced vaccinations fall under the category of unreasonable seizure of your body; or the bodies of your children. They are the epitome of seizure of your being. You should always ask for specific performance from any court in favor of you, the beneficiary of the contract, which is the united states constitution. Contract law states that any contract shall be enforced most favorable in favor of the non-preparer(you). You have a right to claim specific performance of the constitution.

Politicians think they also have the right to do whatever they want during a declared emergency; also a falsehood according to Am. Jurisprudence.

Section 98: Effect of public emergency;

"*While an emergency cannot create power, and* NO
EMERGENCY JUSTIFYS THE VIOLATION OF ANY OF THE
PROVISIONS OF THE UNITED STATES CONSTITUTION OR
STATE CONSTITUTIONS . . . . "

"*On the other hand, a contention that a grave emergency such as
a depression should permit construction of the constitutional provisions
which would meet the emergency was rejected in one case, the court
holding that neither the legislature nor any executive or judicial officer
may disregard the provisions of the constitution in cases of an emergency
where the plain and unequivocal terms of the constitution present no
question of construction as to departures in emergencies.*"

How clear can you get? Even in declared "emergencies," the
spin doctor politicians cannot disregard your constitutional rights.
Nowhere in the constitution does it state that your rights can be
suspended due to any emergency.

More goodies from Am. Jurisprudence:

Section 117:

The courts are not at liberty to search for meanings beyond
the instrument of the constitution. The courts must apply the
terms of the constitution as written.

Section 155:

The courts are not at liberty to overlook or disregard the
constitutional demands. If the constitution prescribes one rule
and the statute another, and a different rule, it is the duty of the
courts to declare that the constitution and not the statute governs
in cases before them for judgment.

Sections 255, 256:

An unconstitutional law is null and wholly void. An
unconstitutional law is null and void from the date of enactment.
No repeal of these unconstitutional laws are necessary. No one is
bound to obey an unconstitutional law.

Sections 257, 258:

On the other hand, it is clear that congress cannot by authorization or ratification give the slightest effect to a state law or constitution which is in conflict with the constitution of the united states.

Religious Freedom

The section following this chapter provides you with different methods of fighting for your common law rights, giving you the power of choosing whether or not to vaccinate your child. Many people whimper under such stress, saying they'd rather vaccinate their kids than have to fight the system. I have also known people who have gone to local courts on the issue and lost, simply because their case was based on asking the *wrong questions*. In America, we have *religious freedom*. Not merely the freedom to practice whatever recognized, *organized* religion we choose. But to practice freely, a religion of **ONE** if we choose to, even if no one in the world has ever heard of our religion before. We can be called the *Church Of The Rabbit In The Moon*, worshipping that fictional character. One of the tenets of this religion is that it forbids vaccines, and if anyone makes you go against that tenet by mandating a vaccine on you or your family, they are violating your rights to freely exercise your religious beliefs granted under the constitution. This is why practically all states have religious exemptions to vaccinations in their laws.

You don't have to have a silly religion like the example above to avoid vaccines. Simply put, your religion is how you choose to relate with God in worship. Under your right to worship freely, granted to you by the constitution *through common law*, you can have your body as part of that worship. Your body *is Gods' temple*. It could be your belief that this body, which was given to you by God, as a divine temple, cannot be altered with man made (and thus inferior) chemicals and mixtures, such as vaccines. It can be the belief in your personal religion that only God made substances will pass through your body and blood stream. It can be your religious belief that only your God given immune system will protect you from "germs" and other "contagions"; that it is a mortal sin to place medical chemicals into your body temple to alter God's perfection. It can be your religious standpoint, that receiving a disease naturally and healing from it naturally, is a necessary part of growing and living in God's world. You should ask anyone who challenges you on this point, *"are you attempting to deny me my constitutional right to religious freedom?"* Some schools I have dealt with in the past have declared personal religions that are not the normal, organized ones we usually hear about, as *"frivolous,"* or *"not a valid religion."* Your next good question should be, *"be so kind as to explain to me the legal definition of a frivolous or valid religion."* Medical and school officials would have to be quite dim-witted if they answered this question, since *ANY ANSWER* would wind up becoming a constitutional violation of your rights, regardless of what is written in your State's vaccination statute.

Another great question to ask anyone attempting to push an oppressive statute on you is, *"are you trying to deny me due process of the law by making a legal determination right now?"* This statement is my favorite *"bureaucrat melter."* Some States have limited the religious exemption to vaccines, writing that the exemption needs to be of a *"well recognized denomination, whose teachings include reliance on prayer or spiritual means alone for healing."* The same limits also require a person to be an adherent member of the religious organization. Now before you run out and join the local Christian Science Church to avoid oppressive vaccines, remember you must learn to be a bulldog when it comes to this issue. The simple wording of religious exemptions such as this, which claim an exemption must be of a specific "well recognized religious denomination," would more than likely be held as unconstitutional by any court, if not totally void primarily for its' vagueness. The good news is that most State vaccine statutes are not written this way. More and more churches as well, are speaking out against compulsory vaccines, so *Keep strong!* By asking the right questions, you will prevail.

I have also formed a religion called, *"The Church of Christ Consciousness."* I have taken the time to be sure all the documents validating this church are in accordance with the guidelines for worship under the constitution of these united states. You can become an *adherent member* of this church at any time. We ask for a one time donation of $25 (US FRN) if you are able. You will receive a packet of detailed information explaining the religious tenets of the church, which include *reliance on prayer or spiritual means alone for healing,* as well as detailed instructions on beating vaccination bureaucracy by standing firm in these religious beliefs. Understand this *does not* mean that you are vowing to never use medicines or other remedies, or attend different religious functions. Part of the prayer practices of this church include receiving inner messages from God, which guide you to the correct therapies to use for yourself and your children *in extreme, life threatening situations only.* Otherwise, these religious tenets do not permit you to use medications, vaccinations, or other remedies as a means of healing. You will receive a document stating that you are *an adherent member of this religious faith*, and yes, you can be an adherent member of two religions at the same time. You don't have to give up any other family religion to be a member of the Church of Christ Consciousness. Further information on becoming involved in this church can be found in the documents section.

It is also important to understand that this issue may very well turn out to be a **HUGE** issue. Regardless of your creator endowed, natural and unalienable rights, most State courts believe that an individual *does not* have absolute freedom from State invasion of his body. This terrible fact is rooted, once again, in the religion of the medical profession that preaches the doctrine of the germ theory. They have convinced politicians and lawmakers at large to adhere to this doctrine, otherwise burn in the eternal damnation of epidemic and contagious disease death rate increases, of which they would be deemed fully responsible. State courts have always ruled, up to this point anyway, that the individual, regardless of religious or other belief, has an obligation to society to help prevent the spread of "contagious" disease. Being a citizen of the State and a member of society thus, you must give up your common law right of freedom from body invasion to some extent for the good of the State. What form of government is this beginning to sound like?

State courts rule time and time again that they have authority over a persons' individual rights, since the rights of the citizens of a State as a group are more important than a single individuals' rights. Therefore, in the event of any "State interest," you and your children can be forcefully medicated with vaccines.

Now it doesn't stop there, otherwise everything we have written thus far is a waste of time. Again, *success in this legal arena all comes down to having a clear mind, keeping calm and asking the right questions. If you can do that, you will avoid going to court all together, without ever having to speak to a lawyer or have your children vaccinated.* Once the right questions are asked, you are backing school and health department professionals in a corner they can only get out of if they answer those questions. *What the medical cartel fears most,* is that these questions could lead to a legal process when brought before a judge, that very possibly could create a *legal precedent* which could change the way courts now look at compulsory vaccines. *This very threat of legal precedent is what keeps you from having to pay a lawyer, go to court and adhere to compulsory vaccine laws.*

The courts have ruled that pharmaceutical companies must adequately warn the consumer of the potentially dangerous propensity of their products. Failure to do so renders their product *"unreasonably dangerous,"* and exposes them to liability for injuries. Warning a doctor alone is not sufficient to relieve the manufacturer from liability, as was so declared by another legal precedent. *The courts have ruled that it is the responsibility of the manufacturer to see that the warnings reach the consumer.* This shows that a warning of potential danger regarding any vaccine, *MUST* reach the patient or parent so that vaccine is not deemed *"unreasonably dangerous."* This can only be done by either your pediatrician directly warning you before administering the shot, or by pamphlet information given directly to you, explaining its' warnings and potential risks. *Legally, it seems quite inconsistent to require a manufacturer of vaccines to warn the consumer of potential risks, and then compel that same consumer to be injected against their will.* This is a very solid legal point.

If the consumer is not allowed to make a choice after knowing the risks, what good are knowing the risks? This is precisely how the government opens itself up to huge liability year after year from vaccine damage. The laws being written in this way absolve the pharmaceutical companies from liability, since by law they gave you fair warning your child could become brain damaged. The State becomes more liable then since they forced you to have the child vaccinated regardless of the warning, and they pay out millions of dollars each year to prove it. All things being as they are, I suspect the laws have been written this way for good reason. The medical cartel is behind the lobbying efforts which engineered this complicated network of legal and medical fraud.

Insurance companies generally refuse to underwrite participation in any compulsory vaccine program. In the 1960's pharmaceutical companies paid out huge judgments for injuries related to single polio vaccines and *Quadrigen,* a four in one vaccine targeted against diphtheria, tetanus, pertussis and polio. Many insurance companies refused coverage for damages related to the "swine flu" vaccine program on this basis alone. Between 1979 and 1983 a staggering 9121 lawsuits were filed against the United States for damages related to swine flu and other vaccines, and $1,150,000 was paid out. As of December 1979 for the swine flu vaccine alone, 3813 administrative claims had been filed for a total of $3,417,000,000 in damages. Of these claims, only 118 were paid! This is merely 3% of the total claims filed, which only paid a total of 2.7 million after settlement! This is a mockery of legal justice and an outrage to society in general. Congress then passed a statute under which the United States accepted liability for injury or death arising out of the administration of the swine flu program. This sealed liability to the U.S. government and absolved the pharmaceutical companies, once again. It sure seems that local, State and federal government wish to be the insurer of the public against injuries or deaths related to vaccines, having some interesting affection for the pharmaceutical companies and a need to protect them from ongoing legal hassles. Interesting indeed. Will the real government for and of the people, please stand up?! Hmmmmm. No one seems to be standing up. Okay then, will the real government masquerading as the government for and of the people please stand up?!

Unconsented medical treatment further constitutes assault and battery, and exposes medical doctors, hospitals and the State to liability for money damages due to such treatment. An individual can decide to live in pain, to shorten her life, or even die rather than submit to medical treatment against her wishes. The courts have ruled that: *"no right is held more sacred, or is more carefully guarded by the common law, than the right of every individual to the possession and control of his own person, free from restraint of interference of others unless by clear and unquestionable authority of law"* (*Union Pacific Railway Co. vs. Botsford*).

An individual according to the State however, *does not* have absolute freedom from invasion of his body. Further, if an individual *does not wish protection under the law from the State,* he may be excused from the law if the rest of society is not hurt by his actions. This is an important point. The State, parroting doctrine from the medical cartel, will insist control over you and your child's bodies to insure neither of you become the next Typhoid Mary. *But if vaccines truly work, and the bulk of society has received them, what does the State have to worry about?* This is a very useful question you should always remember to ask. There could be hundreds of unvaccinated Typhoid Mary's running around, possibly being carriers for other diseases as well. So what! The other members of society have been vaccinated. Vaccines work. Not a problem. Well, this is a huge problem for the State, because *State vaccination programs have never been about protecting the masses from disease.* They are primarily about receiving huge money payoffs, masquerading as *"federal aid"* to promote vaccine programs. The more vaccines a State enforces, the more money it receives. If one person gets out of the pen and starts spreading the news that they are unvaccinated and doing just fine, word will catch on. Then more and more people would choose not to be vaccinated or subject their children to it. Then the State would argue that we would have larger and larger portions of the population becoming ill with contagious disease, but this is another lie. There have never been any studies comparing the overall health and well being of unvaccinated people to vaccinated, and the medical cartel never wants an honest study completed in this arena. To do so would thwart their vaccination profits and control of the people, and further open lawmakers to responsibility for ethically questionable laws which have supported compulsory vaccine programs for decades. *The plain and simple truth is that unvaccinated people, especially children, are far healthier than the vaccinated population at large.*

We as a nation of sovereign people, need to push for a complete moratorium on compulsory vaccines. If this is done, we can effectively study the difference in vaccinated and unvaccinated groups over a long range study. I will guarantee you, and place everything I own on the outcome, that the unvaccinated group will be deemed far healthier.

Most states also provide medical exemptions to vaccination. This is another avenue of relief from the vaccination Gestapo, in that medical exemptions will no doubt always be written into State law to cover the States' liability in court. States realize there are many vaccination related lawsuits begun each year, and people wind up suing the State who they say, forced them to vaccinate their now brain damaged, or dead child. Part of the States' legal defense is always their medical exemption to vaccination, and they will propose that it was your responsibility as the parent to be sure your child was medically fit to receive the vaccine.

Here's how you can make the medical exemption work for you. Send certified letters titled, ***Requests For Assurance Of Medical Treatment and Relief Upon Damage***, (found in the forms section) to your State and town's department of health officials, as well as to any school officials who are blocking your child's entrance due to no vaccines. The letter states that you are willing to comply with the vaccination laws as long as you can be guaranteed the State, town and school will cover any and all possible damages that may occur to your child via the vaccine. The letter also requests a guarantee that the vaccine will prevent the particular disease or diseases for which it is being given. The letter does not ask for a guarantee of *immunity*, because legally and medically all immunity means is that a person shows antibodies in her blood for a particular disease. Immunity is by no means a guarantee of wellbeing, or prevention from any disease. In many cases this letter alone will create enough turmoil to allow your child to return to school without vaccines. To my knowledge, no one in the history of mankind has ever signed such a letter, and the chances for ending any vaccination dilemma with your school are high.

I have also known of people who try and reason with the pediatrician, asking him to please read the packet insert to them so they can understand what they're getting into. This can lead to the MD granting you the medical exemption, but more likely he will attempt to intimidate you. Pediatricians tell you that there is a greater chance of being struck by lightening than in developing those kinds of side effects, printed clearly in the packet insert from the vaccine. Also, all parents should note that the packet inserts *do not* mention that the vaccine will prevent the disease it is given for. It only states that it will increase antibody counts, which you now know are totally worthless.

In some cases, especially with concern to private schools, the *Release From Liability Of Disease* letter in the forms section works quite well. Notarize this letter and hand it to all school officials and doctors afraid of loosing their jobs for not following the law. It places all the emphasis back on you legally for liability in case your child becomes ill, and fully releases the doctor or school from such liability.

Another letter provided in the next section is titled, *Request For Medical Exemption Under State Statute*, and it states that there is enough evidence in valid research on vaccinations to suggest your child is eligible for a medical exemption under the law. They always come back at you and say you need a medical doctor to claim a vaccine medical exemption for your child, and if you have a good relationship with an MD somewhere, this can surely make the process move a lot smoother. If you can't get an MD to sign for a medical exemption, then you are still standing on a strong legal ground at the common law. If they refuse to sign your certified *Request For Assurance Of Medical Treatment and Relief Upon Damage* letter (they would be crazy if they did sign it), as well as refuse you a medical exemption, and yet still block access for your child into school, you are building a case to sue the State, town and school for their actions. Find a lawyer who will support you in this kind of suit. If and when you still have to go to court, your lawyer should be experienced in issues concerning first amendment rights for free exercise of religion. The court always argues that the health of the State population in general will be at risk if certain individuals are allowed to not vaccinate their children. *Your lawyer must be able to prove fully before the court that your decision to not vaccinate can in no way harm society as a whole, especially if vaccinations are truly believed to work and the bulk of school children are vaccinated.* Considering this scenario, I would love to see a court rule that vaccination programs cannot be guaranteed effective. That would open up some very interesting doors for debate.

In any State court case regarding compulsory vaccines, the State's interest (on the books anyway) is the protection of its' citizens from the spread of communicable diseases. It can certainly be argued in the conventional sense, that routine compulsory vaccinations should not be permitted to interfere with your religious rights, since there are at present, no epidemics running amok, and you are not likely to begin one. The party line is indeed, that vaccines have conquered most contagious disease! Whopsie do for that! Since everyone is already safe, why should you have to rescind your religious beliefs of avoiding invasive medical chemicals being injected into your family's blood streams? The immediacy of the health factor for contagious disease is no longer so great an issue. Any dispute the State now puts forth only weakens its' argument supporting compulsory vaccines! After all, if compulsory vaccines have been so great, why worry about you and your family? *The State cannot adequately prove that school children who do not receive vaccines create an immediate or even threatened danger to the other, vaccinated school children, or the public at large, because to do so invalidates the effectiveness of vaccine programs.* A good lawyer can then place the burden on the State to prove a present or threatening danger to the public which can occur as a result of your decision to not vaccinate. If the State does present "expert" witness to defend its' case to vaccinate, then your lawyer could present the true side of the scientific and medical vaccine controversy, well sighted in this book and known to the public eye in 2000. Many "experts" cringe at such truth, and have difficulty maintaining their poise against the enormous challenge of questioned fact regarding compulsory vaccines. If enough cases are presented to the courts in this manner, I feel the States will have to begin ruling more and more in favor of exemption. This of course, means more and more people have to legally challenge compulsory vaccines. Without the action of the people, nothing will get done.

Here is another way the *Request For Assurance Of Medical Treatment and Relief Upon Damage* letter can be used at your pediatricians' office. Go the doctors' office with several witnesses, and ask your pediatrician to sign it, just in case your child becomes ill or gets hurt in any way from the shots. No doctor in their right mind will ever sign it, so you simply walk out with your child and witnesses, and say good-bye. Now you are asking better questions. *You have shifted the issue to a more complex one of attempting to gain assurance for a medical operation, and the possibility of medical mal-practice if the doctor refuses to give you that assurance.* You then send a letter to the State and town departments of health, and the school officials, stating that you attempted to get your child vaccinated as they requested, but the doctor would not vaccinate your child. Have your witnesses write up and notarize affidavits confirming this fact. Send the affidavits along as well (bureaucrats just love affidavits!). They may then tell you to forget about your silly letter of relief and get your child vaccinated anyway. *Remember to ask the right questions always with regards to dealing with these bureaucrats.* You should then mention that you couldn't help but notice that there is a medical exemption to vaccination written within the law. They will acknowledge there indeed is one. Then ask them how one would know if their child falls under this category. They will say your pediatrician has to determine that due to your child's particular sensitivity, or problem which precludes the child from receiving a vaccine. **Here's where you have them!** *If the pediatrician already refused to sign the Request For Assurance Of Medical Treatment and Relief Upon Damage form, she is confirming her uncertainty, professionally and medically, that your child will not be effected adversely by the vaccine. If the* *pediatrician who administers the shot, is not certain enough to sign a form stating your child will not be harmed after the shot, that is your admission from the pediatrician of a medical exemption!* The State can well argue here, that you were attempting to coerce the pediatrician into signing something he could not possibly provide a guarantee for, since the packet inserts of all vaccines do claim certain risks. Whenever a person goes in for an operation, or takes a medicine of any kind, there are also certain risks. But a person *chooses* to take medication and have operations. He may not, as is the case here, choose to have a vaccination.

Making life a lot easier however, is the fact that most states stand by their religious exemption clauses without providing any extra trouble for the parents. There are several religions you may become part of which include anti-vaccination beliefs as religious doctrine. As noted, one such religion is included in the forms section. The problem is usually not with the State, but with some ultra brain washed school nurse or official, who feels they have to save your child from your ill decision making. Again, the best advice is to be a bulldog. Stand firm in what you believe, and know you have God given, creator endowed unalienable rights. When you learn how to exercise your common law rights, this process will become easier and easier.

Another very interesting method of avoiding compulsory vaccines deals with your legal **right to privacy**. This has yet to be used successfully, but the argument has tremendous potential for the future. In court, it can be stated that this right comes from the Bill of Rights, the 9th and 14th amendments. The right to personal privacy is based on the theory that the individual has the right to control his own body, and to make fundamental decisions about his own life. This right extends to children as well. As well as religious exemption, this right is limited by the particular State's compelling interest. The State could be made to show sufficient interest in order to override a person's right to privacy with regards to his decision to not vaccinate. In the past, this right has been used successfully with respect to abortion, euthanasia, drugs to mental patients and making certain kinds of important decisions with respect to one's body. Vaccines are proven to be harmful to the body, and by their very nature are an assault on the body. There is always the risk of dangerous side effects as noted by the manufacturer. If the decision to be vaccinated or not falls within the control over one's body, it is therefore protected by the constitutional right of privacy. State prosecutors would be hard pressed to meet the burden of proof, showing a State interest compelling enough to override the fundamental right to privacy. In this case, they would be required to show that a child who was not vaccinated would be presenting a great risk to her health. Given the ever mounting public evidence demonstrating the exact opposite, this would be extremely difficult for a prosecutor to do. *Remember, the party line is that public health has improved vastly from the time these laws were first passed, and vaccines are the heroes!* If a prosecutor agues this party line, he is again going against the vaccination claim to fame, and most courts do not want to open those doors.

Playing the legal chess game in this way is very important. The majority of people are vaccinated today because they want to be, and they believe vaccines keep their children healthy (much like a good blood letting!). The majority of people then, by the popular vote, are fully protected from the wonders of vaccine technology. Surely society cannot be harmed if a certain segment of the population chooses to object to, and refrain from vaccines.

Another way to understand the common law, is to realize that you have many other rights, granted to you by God alone, that *the constitution of these united states* cannot infringe upon. Most Americans believe their rights are granted them by the bill of rights and the constitution primarily, but this is not how our country was formed. First and foremost, you have God given, creator endowed unalienable rights to pure health and happiness, and to be a sovereign without subjects in your own home. The ninth and tenth amendments to the constitution confirm this fact;

" . . . the enumeration in the constitution of certain rights shall not be construed to deny or disparage others [other rights] retained by the people . . . . the powers not delegated to the united states by the constitution, are reserved to the states respectively or to the people . . . . "

The 14th amendment reads;

"Neither slavery nor involuntary servitude shall exist in the United States or any place subject to its' jurisdiction."

In reading this amendment, one has to wonder why "slavery" and "involuntary servitude" are distinguished from one another. Any idea why? They seem like the same thing, but they are very different. Involuntary servitude is placed in the 14th amendment to distinguish it from *"voluntary servitude,"* which is the basis of any **legal contract under commercial law.** Just so you know, under United States commercial law, whenever you sign a contract you waive all your rights, and are now bound by the contents of the contractual agreement you signed. What kinds of contracts have you become involved in without prior knowledge? There are many, so to save time we'll focus on the one that relates to compulsory vaccinations, and that is a **marriage license.** A typical State marriage license reads;

"The State is a party to every marriage contract of its' own residence, as well as the guardians of its' morals."

Every marriage license is thus an agreement to a *three way* legal marriage between the husband, the wife and the State. All children of these types of marriages are thus wards of the State as well as children of the marriage. So now your child goes to a State funded public school, and they say *no shots, no school.* The State can rule that due to your marriage contract, it has an equal say in the welfare of your children. You have to consider the State thus in all the vital decision making processes you make as parents. What form of government does this sound like?

Does this particular marriage contract mean that if you don't comply with vaccination laws, the State will come into your home and forcefully vaccinate you and your children? Probably not now, but this is a real possibility for the future unless public awareness of vaccination fraud increases. Public awareness has become the primary motivation for writing this book . . . . God only knows I won't get rich from it.

The marriage contract does constitute a three party contract with the State the couple resides in, and it entitles the couple to certain "privileges" under State law, such as the privilege to send your children to a public school. Part of exercising this privilege however, is to follow your States laws and vaccinate your children. After all, they are one third the ward of the State. A State cannot deny a married couple their common law rights (as long as the exercise of those rights does not harm anyone else), but a State can deny a married couple a privilege. This is the legal basis for the no shots, no school issue. If the State finds you in any way a "bad parent," they can also walk in through the DCF, and remove your children from your home. I agree that in some cases, children do need to be removed from abusive environments, and in this capacity the DCF is necessary. Where is the line drawn however? Who decided where that line is? We do as a people, but if we don't speak up, they will decide for us.

Why is all this happening?

I have a brother who once said to me that conspiracies like this could never happen, because they would be discovered and printed all over the grand media and broadcasted on every TV channel. Well, I wish this were truly how our world works today, but as many of you realize, this is just not so. The United States *"free"* press and media print and broadcast whatever party line they are instructed to print and broadcast. In the rare case that something of truth really does reach a special prime time news show, it is only for a short segment. People soon forget or fall back onto a psychological state of denial and disbelief called, *"that just can't be."*

I only wish the material presented in this book were not true. Over the years I have been compiling research on the subject, I have gone through an array of emotions and states of denial, only to be presented with more and more blatant evidence. The fact that vaccines create cancer, autism and other degenerative neurological disorders is so blatantly obvious from the perspectives of both science and law, that the issue is no longer up for debate.

This very real health threat, pandemic by it's own creation, will render *most* of the world's population complete with neurological and varying levels of brain dysfunction within the next few decades if we do not put a stop to it now. That means *RIGHT NOW!*

Many people over the years have asked me how and why this all could be happening. These are very good questions that everyone should start with. From all my research on the subject, I offer to you 3 *possible* scenarios as an answer:

1) **The most obvious,** and the primary premise of this book, is common *greed.* A complex strata of people too busy to look at the facts because they are too busy counting profits, as well as figuring new ways to avoid litigation and create new profits. Blinded by their holy cash cow, they refuse to see how the germ theory and all it's by-products, like vaccines, are destroying the very core of civilization. They hear the statistics on cancer and autism, and do everything they can to deny any correlation to vaccines and other medications simply because of their love of money. Even though they promote vaccines on all other children, the smart ones within the system reaping the profits will not vaccinate their own kids because they really do know better. Mark my word on that.

2) **The most unlikely,** is that they really believe they are doing good, fervently believe what they have been told about the germ theory, and are just too stubborn to think otherwise. I have pondered this premise quite a bit over the past decade, and with each year it becomes more and more ridiculous due to overwhelming evidence to the contrary. I do believe however, that many medical doctors fall into this category.

3) **The most frightening, however quite possible scenario,** is a conspiracy of a number of individuals in mega power positions around the globe, most likely organized together in some fashion to control the masses of the Earth's population for their sole benefit. Obviously, we would be referring to the Illuminati in this scenario. Numerous reports over the past 4 decades suggest the presence within government and other

powerful organizations, of a *demonic like* faction that has become ever present. With carefully planned precision to it's movements and goals, this faction has secretly operated within many government agencies for years, most likely with its' ultimate goal to consume all. The members of this faction know vaccines and other medical programs are totally counterproductive to Human existence, and they have planned it that way. They believe the *other* people of the world are inferior, and use *them* for whatever purposes suit their benefit. They use the venues of mandatory vaccine programs, and their influence to enforce police power on such mandates, for massive genetic experiments, population control by inducing illness, the intentional altering of brain activity for mind control, the intentional creation of brain damage in children, so *select* populations of people never get too smart to claim any true power for themselves, and even genocide of certain populations if they deem necessary. Does anyone really know what is in those shots? It has never ceased to amaze me that parents allow their children, the most precious aspects of their lives, to be injected with substances they know nothing about. If this does not change, *and fast,* mankind can very well be subject to extinction at the will of whatever group of people decide to *"rule the world."* This may sound like science fiction folks, but I assure you, I have not overdosed on the *"X-Files."* This scenario can be very real.

One should seriously consider, in today's world, the reality of scenario #3 above. The pharmaceutical industry is owned and controlled by the same conglomerate corporate mobsters that are attempting to keep you, and your children, in slavery. This industry is completely unregulated. Any pseudo *"regulation"* from any agency which has a vested financial interest in selling vaccines and drugs (for example, the FDA) is similar to the fox being granted regulatory authority over the hen house. It's all a game, and they assume you are just too stupid, too afraid, too busy, too addicted, or too sick to know what they are really doing. So, it continues . . . .

Do you really believe this vaccine and drug industry has your best interest in mind? Do you really believe they respect the sanctity or your children and act first in their best interest? It is all a fairy tale.

It is, in reality, more likely that this conglomerate has a tremendous agenda of control in mind for your life and the lives of your future generations. Control of your financial world via bogus "laws" via IRC 26, the impossible to decipher Internal Revenue Code. Control of your mind through a never ending bombardment of images, sounds, phrases and manufactured "emergencies," all carefully designed to turn you into Pavlov's dog. Control of your diet through the introduction of hundreds of addictive chemicals and other additives into the manufactured food supply.

And now, control of your body through the constant onslaught of injected chemicals via vaccines, or oral chemicals in the case of "medications." Is it really so far fetched, paranoid, and/or "conspiracy minded," to believe that rather than benevolence, they actually have a malevolent agenda in mind which would include the following;

1. The intentional addition of carcinogens, and other poisons to vaccines to keep a constant level of disease in any chosen population for profit.

2. The intentional addition of "slow killer" poisons, into the vaccines of any given population that has been selected for genocide.

3. The intentional addition of brain toxins into children's vaccines, placed there to purposely render future generations more dull intellectually, and more passive to any purported authority. In essence, to ensure that future generations are more autonomous, less creative, and obedient worker robots for the *"good of the state."*

4. The seeding of select populations with disease creating micro-chips, able to create a certain disease at a certain time in life.

5. The addition of micro-chips that lay dormant and undetected, but can be activated via satellite at any time to spontaneously end the life of any human being who becomes a problem to the "state."

6. The addition of micro-chips that emit a unique carrier frequency for each human being, used as a tracking device able to locate anyone via satellite.

We, as a race of beings, need to stand up immediately and realize that these scenarios are not mere science fiction. In today's greedy technological nightmare of a world, these scenarios are quite possible. When you consider all the facts, you can deduce from logic that they are even, quite probable. We need to stand together in our power and ask good questions, while we still have power and the ability to use our voices. I have faith that things can change for the better, but I am certain they will not unless more and more people wake up. My sole intention for writing this book is to help you wake up, so that, hopefully, you will wake up someone else. Then, hopefully, they may wake up someone else, and then hopefully . . . . It is my prayer and constant vision that we all grow someday to understand the full meaning, and responsibility of true sovereignty and freedom. Greed, and the greedy, must perish.

Clarence Darrow, the defending attorney for the school teacher in the famous *"Scopes monkey trial"* in 1925, is one of my all time favorite Americans (and played very well by Jack Lemmon in the new version of *"Inherit The Wind."* Rent it!). He had this to say of the medical profession [cartel] back in the 1930's;

"The efforts of the medical profession in the United States to control the treatment of human ailments is not due to its' love of humanity. It is due to its' love of its' job, which it proposes to monopolize. It has been carrying on a vigorous campaign all over the country against new methods of schools of healing, because it wants [all] the business, and insists that nobody shall live or die without its' services. Whether it cures more or fewer people than schools which do not use medicines, or whether it cures anybody at all, are debatable questions which I shall not attempt to discuss. I stand for everybody's right to regulate their own life, so long as it doesn't infringe on other peoples' rights to do the same. If a man

wants to live or die without the aid of the medical profession, he should be permitted to do so. If he hasn't this right, it is pretty hard to tell what right he should have.

Now I would have no argument with the medical profession if they would leave me alone. I am willing that they should advertise their wares, but I object to being forced to patronize them. They have specifics [vaccines] to prevent one from catching almost every disease, yet not one of them can explain how the prevention is brought about. Nor can he prove that it does prevent. They are not content to vaccinate [only] those who apply to them, but they ask the State to compel everyone to be vaccinated. I might as well ask the State to compel everyone to hire me to try their law cases. Sometime, if they keep on, and they will keep on if the people give them the chance, they will be able to vaccinate us for everything, and we shall be compelled to submit. I have watched this medical profession for a long time, and it bears watching, and I know that there is not a single thing effecting human life that they will not lay their hands on if we give them the chance."

What a perfect ending to this text. Nothing says it better. Learn your rights and exercise them well before it's too late, and you loose all of them. Remember, stating it clearly about the true nature of law (or lawlessness) today, is this. *If people do not know their rights, then they have none.* This medical cartel is looking to consume every aspect of our lives, and only the people, empowered with the truth of their sovereign rights to freedom, can stop them. There is still time to stop them, and I urge everyone reading this text to reach out, speak out, share what they have learned, and move forward. It can be done. I've got one more quote to repeat for you from Winston Churchill;

"It is better to fight, when there is little chance of winning, then to have to fight when there is no chance at all . . . ."

God bless America. God bless us all.

Forms and References

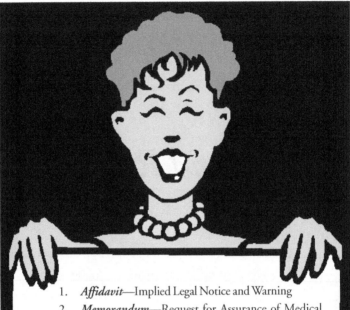

1. *Affidavit*—Implied Legal Notice and Warning
2. *Memorandum*—Request for Assurance of Medical Treatment and Relief Upon Damage
3. *Affidavit* of Probable Cause for Attempted Assault and Battery
4. *Affidavit*—Release from Liability of Disease
5. *Memorandum*—Request for Medical Exemption under State statute
6. Request For Access To Documents Under your State's *Freedom of Information act*
7. Church of Christ Consciousness Information
8. *Hospital Zinger Affidavit* (if they say they can force you to have your newborn vaccinated or medicated): *NOTICE of Patient and New Parents Rights to Refuse Medical Treatments After Childbirth*
9. *PUBLIC RECORDS ACT ZINGER*: For school "officials" that are giving you trouble.

Please note: this section does not contain any legal advice. It contains only law research for your continued education.

This section will provide you with the necessary forms as dictated by the last chapter. It has been my experience that if your paperwork is done properly, and timely, you can toss any vaccination mongrel right out the window, get your kids into school and sue any lawyer for damages if he gets in your way.

There are a few things to understand before you get started.

1. You are not going to sue, or file paperwork *"in the system."* When we say *"in the system,"* we are talking about within the confines of **statutory law.** Those federal and state statutory courts **ARE NOT YOUR COURTS.** Statutory law and courts are for corporations and corporate fictions, or corporate trusts (like your ALL CAPS NAME). You may **volunteer** to go into those statutory courts, and give up your common law jurisdiction if you choose. But why would you do this? It is certainly more common for lawyers and judges to coerce you into showing up in their courts by lying and using fear tactics. This is how they gain jurisdiction over you without you knowing what is really going on. When you show up in their courts, you are essentially saying, "okay, I waive my common law unalienable rights and succumb to your will and whim." When you agree to let statutory law have jurisdiction over you, you have absolutely *NO RIGHTS.* When you claim your sovereignty under the common law, you are the master, and they, your servants. *You do this by asking the right questions at the right time.*

All of your paperwork and subsequent filings with your town clerks office, are going to become real by the power of your own sovereignty as an American, and under the *COMMON LAW, which is your law.* You can only claim this if you **ARE NOT** represented by a BAR card attorney (a regular lawyer). I have yet to see a lawyer in any state that wanted to get involved with this kind of sovereignty paperwork.

2. The concept of a *"license to practice law"* does not exist, by any real sense, in any state that I have found thus far in my research. In essence, the supposed *law license* is a fiction. All graduates of law schools are eligible to take a state **BAR (The term "BAR" is an acronym for British Accredited Registry)** EXAMINATION. See: **http://www.healthfreedom.info/ BAR%20Association.htm** If they pass, they receive what is known as a **BAR CARD** for that particular states' **BAR ASSOCIATION.** A BAR card is nothing more than a membership into a club of graduated lawyers who have passed the exam. The BAR card itself has *NEVER* been demonstrated anywhere legally to be a license to practice law. Yet, people get thrown into jail for practicing law without a license. How is this possible, when lawyers do not even have a license to practice law? Ask the next lawyer you come across and watch her dance. A very powerful question to ask of a lawyer who is bothering you, especially in writing, is for that lawyer to demonstrate their license to practice law and make legal determinations. This can get extremely amusing.

3. When you make your AFFIDAVITS, understand that they can contain no conjecture, and only facts. It is also best to keep them clear of any statutory law you may assume you know. An Affidavit is simply a sworn statement of FACTS. You are stating, to the best of your knowledge and ability, that these events occurred on these dates, and therefore you can draw certain conclusions and claim damages if necessary. An un-rebutted Affidavit stands as truth in the common law, and in commerce. This means that if a lawyer or judge does not answer the Affidavit you have filed with the town clerks' office against

them, in what is known as a *"counter-affidavit," than everything in your original Affidavit stands as truth.* They must answer each claim against them in your original Affidavit to the letter. If they miss one, or simply only answer what they feel like answering and leave the rest, the same truth applies. Your original Affidavit stands as truth. If they are totally non-responsive, your original Affidavit stands as truth after 30 days. This means you can state, "Mrs. Brainwashed, school nurse at Federal Public Elementary school, and their school lawyer, Mr. Whimpie, failed to show me proof that the statutory vaccination laws of the state of New York actually apply to me or my son. She is denying my son access to school and thus causing me and my family a damage." When they do not rebutt this claim, you win! Send your kid to school and expect that they will accept him. Always have a witness with you. If they do not let him come into the school, file a criminal complaint Affidavit with the town and local sheriff's office, and begin billing the school $1000 a day for your damages. Send the bill weekly if necessary. In extreme examples, if your child has still not been allowed to attend school, begin a commercial lien process to collect your damages. *DESM can help you with this process (954-934-0304).*

4. Some town clerks offices will give you trouble when filing your Affidavits or other related paperwork for your claim of sovereignty. Simply ask, *"where do I file Affidavits and other documents for public record?"* If they are still not willing to help, ask, *"are you making a legal determination right now?"* They have to give you an answer. If they do not, they are causing you a damage. As well, judges and/or lawyers do not have any authority to upset, alter, or in any way change what is already in public record. Only YOU can remove what you have placed in public record. If necessary, you need to stand firm in these truths.

5. The paperwork which follows can work in this manner. You are going to be making claims and statements that you believe are true and correct, and you are going to send these

claims in paper form to the people who are bothering you, or otherwise blocking your child's entrance into school. Since they are causing you a damage, you are simply asking them why they are doing this when you know the truth is _____. You are then going to insist that they state their authority to do what they are doing in many different ways.

6. When they do not answer you, or answer you in an aberrant or unresponsive manner, you then file an Affidavit, now stating that those questions you asked of them are now all true. In other words, you initially ask them to prove that the vaccine laws apply to you, and for their license to practice law. If they do not provide you with a suitable answer in a counter-affidavit form, then your Affidavit will state "Mr. Jones has no authority to block my child from school. The vaccination laws of this state do not apply to me. Mr. Jones does not have a license to practice law." If a lawyer does not have a license to practice law, shouldn't that be considered practicing law without a license?

If, after knowing all this, you decide you do have to go to court, you may want to consider going on your own; what is known as *Pro Se*. If you appear Pro Se in the court room, you are demonstrating to the court that you are appearing *Sui juris*, another legal term which means, according to *Black's Law Dictionary*, "*appearing in one's own right; possessing full social and civil rights; not under any legal disability, or the power of another, or guardianship; having capacity to manage one's own affairs; not under legal disability to act for one's self.*" Sui juris simply means *in your own right, with no higher title confining you.* In other words, you are in the courtroom on your own, of sound mind and body, complete with all your common law rights because you have not waived them under any particular contract.

In contrast, whenever you go to court with a lawyer, the lawyer speaks for you, and you waive your common law rights to the court. An unfortunate technicality of approaching the courtroom represented by an attorney, is that the lawyer's first obligation is not to you. She is first an officer of the court, which is her primary allegiance, and must uphold the statutory law over your rights and concerns. Again, you should only go with an attorney (BAR card lawyer) if you absolutely do not feel you can handle this process on your own. You may still be able to accomplish something with a lawyer, but you are going to be bound by whatever is within the statutory law. *I do however, recommend retaining the services of a lawyer competent in vaccination issues if you feel you can get what you want in this way, if the statutory laws may run in your favor.*

Another option is retaining the services of a competent lawyer, or law student, to help you prepare your Pro Se case. If you have the time, learning how to present a case Pro Se is a marvelous learning experience. You have to make it known that these particular State vaccination statutes do not apply to you, and that you are in no way harming anyone by choosing not to vaccinate.

These forms, coupled with the knowledge in this book, should provide you with all you need to legally avoid vaccinations. The first objective of these forms is to avoid court all together, primarily by counter intimidation of the same bureaucrats who are trying to intimidate you into receiving vaccinations against your will. For further reading on presenting your case Pro Se, obtain the books listed under the *law research* portion of the References section which follows. Remember, be a bulldog, and good luck!

Your Address and date:

Addressed to:

CERTIFIED MAIL #_____

Affidavit

IMPLIED LEGAL NOTICE AND WARNING:

I _____, hereby declare on this day my objection to (being forcefully medicated) (my child being forcefully medicated) due to _____ state's vaccination statute. The reasons for this objection are hereby listed in order:

1. No vaccine can be deemed totally safe, since warnings of many symptoms and disorders arising from a vaccine can be found within the packet inserts of all vaccines the State requires by mandate.

2. The State of _____ has not presented me with any personal guarantee, written or otherwise, that myself or my child will NOT be harmed by said vaccines the State has mandated.

3. Dr._____, who would be administering the vaccines, has not presented me with any personal guarantee, written or otherwise, that myself or my child will NOT be harmed by said vaccines the State has mandated.

4. The following school officials in order (list them all), who are blocking entrance of my child to school until such vaccines are administered, have not presented me

with any personal guarantee, written or otherwise, that my child will NOT be harmed by said vaccines the State has mandated.

5. A listing of valid research, stating that the vaccinations mandated by the State of _____ are linked to disorders such as autism, mental retardation, ADHD, decreased intelligence, cancer, disorders of the skin, allergies, disorders of the eyes and ears, sudden infant death syndrome, Parkinson's disease, dementia, Alzheimer's disease, respiratory and cardiac failure, chronic nervous system dysfunction, meningitis, encephalopathy, seizures, anemia, and epilepsy to name but a few, is included with this Implied Legal Notice.

6. The said vaccinations mandated by the State of _____ do not guarantee that myself or my child will not acquire the diseases in which they claim to prevent.

7. There is no state of emergency regarding any of the diseases the State of _____ is attempting to control with the vaccinations mandated.

8. Since the majority of the population of the State of _____ is vaccinated by their own choice for themselves and their children, if it is truly the position of the State that the vaccinations mandated do control the spread of the diseases they are given for, then my choice not to vaccinate myself or my child cannot possibly create any harm to the vaccinated population.

9. Since the majority of the population of the State of _____ is vaccinated by their own choice for themselves and their children, if it is truly the position of the State that the vaccinations mandated do control the spread of the diseases they are given for, then my choice not to vaccinate myself or my child cannot possibly create an epidemic of any kind that poses a risk to the other citizens of the State.

10. The State of _____ cannot adequately prove that I am placing myself, or my child in danger of acquiring a disease by my choice to not vaccinate, since to date there have been few scientific studies on the general health of unvaccinated persons, vs. the general health of vaccinated ones, within any given population. Private research groups have studied the general health of select unvaccinated people, and the results are that unvaccinated people are generally healthier than the vaccinated population.

11. I am of sound mind and body, and reserve all my common law rights to non-invasion of my body, or my child's body, to chemicals being injected into us that we do not approve of, or agree with.

12. I am of sound mind and body, and reserve all my common law rights to make all the decisions regarding the direction of my life, and the direction of the life (lives) of my child (children), especially with regard to their safety, emotional and physical well-being.

13. I reserve all my rights under the *uniform commercial code,* particularly UCC 1-201 and UCC 3-501, and hereby rescind any and all contracts I may have signed with the State of _____, which caused me to unknowingly waive any of my common law rights, or rights granted to me under the constitution of the united states of America, particularly my first amendment right to religious freedom, and my ninth and tenth amendment rights to have my "*other*" rights not denied or disparaged, and protected under the common law.

14. I am of sound mind and body, and it is my firm philosophical belief that the said vaccinations mandated by the State of _____, have been proven by science to be extremely harmful to my body, or my child's body. Under this belief, and the belief that said mandated vaccinations will create harm to myself or my child, I hereby refuse such vaccines to be entered

into my body or the body of my child without my permission and against my will.

15. I am of sound mind and body, and it is my firm religious belief, following the doctrine of the well organized religion called, _____, that the said vaccinations mandated by the State of _____, are in direct violation of my organized religious beliefs. If I am compelled to have these vaccinations injected into my body, or the body of my child, against my will, the State is violating my first amendment right to religious freedom. I have also enclosed a copy of the tenets of my religion, which prevent me and my child from receiving said vaccinations.

16. I reserve all my legal rights to privacy granted to me under the Bill of Rights, the ninth and fourteenth amendments of the constitution of the united states of America. This right to privacy includes my right to control my own body, and the body of my child, and to make fundamental decisions about my life or the life of my child. Vaccines are harmful to the body, and by their very nature are an assault on the body. There is always a risk of dangerous side effects following the administration of the State of _____ mandated vaccines, as is noted by the manufacturer of said vaccines. I further declare that my right, and my child's right to privacy is fundamental at the common law, especially when the State cannot prove that my decision to not vaccinate myself or my child will in any way harm anyone, or create a potential risk to anyone.

17. I reserve all my constitutional rights, and my rights granted to me under the common law, and herby confirm that I will prosecute the fullest extent of the law if these rights are violated in any way as a result of my decision not to vaccinate.

Sincerely,

STATE OF _____)
)ss
COUNTY OF _____)

BEFORE ME, the undersigned authority, _____,
known to me (or satisfactorily proven) to be the persons whose
names are subscribed to the foregoing instrument, personally
appeared and acknowledged to me that they executed the same as
their free act and deed for the purposes and considerations herein
expressed and the capacity stated, ant that the statements contained
herein are true and correct to the best of their information,
knowledge, and belief.

Subscribed and sworn to before me this____day of ____, 19____.

IN WITNESS WHEREOF, I have set my hand and official seal:

_____
Notary Public

_____ County, _____
My commission Expires:_____

NOTARY SEAL:

Your name, address and date here

Addressed to:

CERTIFIED MAIL #_____

Memorandum in Law
Requests For Assurance of Medical Treatment and Relief Upon Damage(s)

Dear (doctor, school, health department official or department of children and families official):

The State of _____ by statue has mandated that my child (or myself) receive a battery of vaccinations. By their very nature, these vaccinations cannot be guaranteed completely safe without the risk of serious side effects, and / or the development of certain disorders, which include autism, mental retardation, ADHD, decreased intelligence, cancer, disorders of the skin, allergies, disorders of the eyes and ears, sudden infant death syndrome, Parkinson's disease, dementia, Alzheimer's disease, respiratory and cardiac failure, chronic nervous system dysfunction, meningitis, encephalopathy, seizures, anemia, and epilepsy to name but a few. The possibilities of acquiring side effects and any one of these conditions is made very clear by the packet insert, provided by the manufacturer of each vaccine, and packaged with the vaccine itself.

It is also a violation of my philosophical and religious beliefs to receive such toxic chemicals into my bloodstream, or the bloodstream of my child.

However, I am told by medical professionals, as well as school and government officials, that despite all this I am still required by law to be vaccinated against my will and better judgment, or to have my child vaccinated against my will and better judgment. I am also told that these shots in the form of vaccines will provide a level of health for myself or my child that will prevent the disease(s) for which they are administered to prevent.

I sincerely wish to comply with any laws which are found to apply to me, however I cannot at the same time, allow my basic, most fundamental rights granted to me under the common law and the constitution of the united states of America, to be violated. I must be sure that by complying with such vaccination laws mandated by the State of _____, that I will not be forcefully caused to injure myself, or my precious child, by partaking in such action.

I therefore look for you to help in this matter. Since you administer these vaccines on a daily basis to many people (in the case of a doctor), or since you have been following the procedures of the State of _____ vaccination laws for some time (in the case of a school, health department or DCF official), you must have some knowledge, training or insight into the matter that a layman such as myself does not possess.

I wish to trust this knowledge you must possess, which enables you to be sure that the risks to myself or my child are low, and enables you to ethically continue administering these vaccines (in the case of a doctor), or to ethically continue enforcing and supporting such vaccination laws.

Therefore, by signing this form, I am requesting assurance from you that this medical treatment of administering vaccinations will not harm myself or my child in any way, mentally or physically. Also, by signing this form, you are assuring me that myself or my child will have greater health as a result of receiving such mandatory vaccines, and that the vaccines will indeed prevent the disease(s) in which they are administered to prevent. In the event that, by me following the said vaccination laws of the State of _____, myself or my child is damaged mentally or physically in any way, by signing this form you are assuring relief of such damages from your malpractice insurance or private funds (in the case of a doctor), or from some government agency insurance coverage or your own private funds (in the case of a school, health department or DCF official).

Since it is your firm belief that vaccinations create health, and prevent the spread of disease, I am thus asking for your assurance that they will indeed create greater health for me and my child, and that the said vaccinations will not cause any further disorders or diseases to me or my child.

Upon your assurance of these facts by the signing of this notice below, I will subject myself, or my child to the vaccinations.

I,_____, being of sound mind and body, agree to the conditions of this form, *Request for Assurance of Medical treatment and Relief Upon Damage*, that _____ will not be harmed in any way as a result of receiving such vaccinations. I maintain this view because it is my sincere belief that these vaccinations are completely safe, and they enhance the health and well-being of the person who receives them by making that person better able to be resistant to the disease the particular vaccination is given for.

This form can either be notarized or signed with witnesses at the particular office it is being presented in.

Signed, this _____day of _____, (year)_____

Print name _____

Signature _____

Witness _____

Witness_____Witness _____

Addressed to:

CERTIFIED MAIL #_____

Affidavit of Probable Cause
for Attempted Assault and Battery

This is to inform (individuals name, doctor or person at health department or DCF) that your actions concerning the forced vaccination of myself or my child against my will and better judgment constitute a *Probable Cause for Attempted Assault and Battery*. I intend to prosecute you for this action to the fullest extent of the law for the reasons provided:

(In this section, state the particular set of circumstances which occurred with the particular individual. Be sure to include dates and times).

Vaccination, especially a set of vaccinations, are considered a medical operation. I can not authorize such a procedure due to it's highly suspicious nature, and high chance of risk to my greater well-being, or the greater well-being of my child. The reasons for this are as follows:

> No vaccine can be deemed totally safe, since warnings of
> many symptoms and disorders arising from a vaccine can be
> found within the packet inserts of all vaccines the State
> requires by mandate.

The State of _____ has not presented me with any personal guarantee, written or otherwise, that myself or my child will NOT be harmed by said vaccines the State has mandated.

Dr._____, who would be administering the vaccines, has not presented me with any personal guarantee, written or otherwise, that myself or my child will NOT be harmed by said vaccines the State has mandated.

The following school officials in order (list them all), who are blocking entrance of my child to school until such vaccines are administered, have not presented me with any personal guarantee, written or otherwise, that my child will NOT be harmed by said vaccines the State has mandated.

A listing of valid research, stating that the vaccinations mandated by the State of _____ are linked to disorders such as autism, mental retardation, ADHD, decreased intelligence, cancer, disorders of the skin, allergies, disorders of the eyes and ears, sudden infant death syndrome, Parkinson's disease, dementia, Alzheimer's disease, respiratory and cardiac failure, chronic nervous system dysfunction, meningitis, encephalopathy, seizures, anemia, and epilepsy to name but a few, is included with this Implied Legal Notice.

The said vaccinations mandated by the State of _____ do not guarantee that myself or my child will not acquire the diseases in which they claim to prevent.

There is no state of emergency regarding any of the diseases the State of _____ is attempting to control with the vaccinations mandated.

Since the majority of the population of the State of _____ is vaccinated by their own choice for themselves and their children, if it is truly the position of the State that the vaccinations mandated do control the spread of the diseases they are given for, then my choice not to vaccinate myself or my child cannot possibly create any harm to the vaccinated population.

Since the majority of the population of the State of _____ is vaccinated by their own choice for themselves and their children, if it is truly the position of the State that the vaccinations mandated do control the spread of the diseases they are given for, then my choice not to vaccinate myself or my child cannot possibly create an epidemic of any kind that poses a risk to the other citizens of the State.

The State of _____cannot adequately prove that I am placing myself, or my child in danger of acquiring a disease by my choice to not vaccinate, since to date there have been few scientific studies on the general health of unvaccinated persons, vs. the general health of vaccinated ones, within any given population. Private research groups have studied the general health of select unvaccinated people, and the results are that unvaccinated people are generally healthier than the vaccinated population.

I am of sound mind and body, and reserve all my common law rights to non-invasion of my body, or my child's body, to chemicals being injected into us that we do not approve of, or agree with.

I am of sound mind and body, and reserve all my common law rights to make all the decisions regarding the direction of my life, and the direction of the life (lives) of my child (children), especially with regard to their safety, emotional and physical well-being.

I reserve all my rights under the *uniform commercial code,* particularly UCC 1-201 and UCC 3-501, and hereby rescind any and all contracts I may have signed with the State of _____, which caused me to unknowingly waive any of my common law rights, or rights granted to me under the constitution of the united states of America, particularly my first amendment right to religious freedom, and my ninth and tenth amendment rights to have my *"other"* rights not denied or disparaged, and protected under the common law.

I am of sound mind and body, and it is my firm philosophical belief that the said vaccinations mandated by the State of _____, have been proven by science to be extremely harmful to my body, or my child's body. Under this belief, and the belief that said mandated vaccinations will create harm to myself or my child, I hereby refuse such vaccines to be entered into my body or the body of my child without my permission and against my will.

I am of sound mind and body, and it is my firm religious belief, following the doctrine of the well organized religion called, _____, that the said vaccinations mandated by the State of _____, are in direct violation of my organized religious beliefs. If I am compelled to have these vaccinations injected into my body, or the body of my child, against my will, the State is violating my first amendment right to religious freedom. I have also enclosed a copy of the tenets of my religion, which prevent me and my child from receiving said vaccinations.

I reserve all my legal rights to privacy granted to me under the Bill of Rights, the ninth and fourteenth amendments of the constitution of the united states of America. This right to privacy includes my right to control my own body, and the body of my child, and to make fundamental decisions about my life or the life of my child. Vaccines are harmful to the body, and by their very nature are an assault on the body. There is always a risk of dangerous side effects following the administration of the State of _____ mandated vaccines, as is noted by the manufacturer of said vaccines. I further declare that my right, and my child's right to privacy is fundamental at the common law, especially when the State cannot prove that my decision to not vaccinate myself or my child will in any way harm anyone, or create a potential risk to anyone.

I reserve all my constitutional rights, and my rights granted to me under the common law, and herby confirm that I will prosecute to the fullest extent of the law if these rights are violated in any way as a result of my decision not to vaccinate.

If you continue to harass me about receiving or administering such vaccinations against my will and better judgment, or if I or any member of my family are vaccinated by force due to any State vaccination statute or perception by any member of the DCF, I will fully prosecute _____ (name of person or persons involved) and any person who administers such a vaccine for assault and battery under the fullest extent of the law.

Sincerely,

STATE OF _____)
)ss
COUNTY OF _____)

BEFORE ME, the undersigned authority, _____,
known to me (or satisfactorily proven) to be the persons whose
names are subscribed to the foregoing instrument, personally
appeared and acknowledged to me that they executed the same as
their free act and deed for the purposes and considerations herein
expressed and the capacity stated, ant that the statements contained
herein are true and correct to the best of their information,
knowledge, and belief.

Subscribed and sworn to before me this____day of_____, 19____.

IN WITNESS WHEREOF, I have set my hand and official seal:

_____
Notary Public

_____ County, _____
My commission Expires:_____

NOTARY SEAL:

Your name, address and date here

Going to:

CERTIFIED MAIL #_____

Affidavit
Release from Liability of Disease

Dear (doctor, school official or government employee):

I,_____, hereby release you in all ways, legal and otherwise, from any liability or blame that may occur if I, or my child becomes ill to *any extent* with a disease as a result of not receiving the State of _____mandated vaccinations.

I as a parent (or individual) of sound mind and body release and totally indemnify you from any claim, fault, liability or blame which may occur as a result of my decision to not vaccinate myself or my child for any particular disease, whether or not such vaccines are mandated by State law. I assume full responsibility for any consequences, legal or otherwise, that follows as a result of my decision to not vaccinate myself, or _____ (child's name).

Signed this _____ day of _____, (year) _____

Printed name _____

Signature _____

STATE OF _____)
)ss
COUNTY OF _____)

BEFORE ME, the undersigned authority, _____,
known to me (or satisfactorily proven) to be the persons whose
names are subscribed to the foregoing instrument, personally
appeared and acknowledged to me that they executed the same as
their free act and deed for the purposes and considerations herein
expressed and the capacity stated, ant that the statements contained
herein are true and correct to the best of their information,
knowledge, and belief.

Subscribed and sworn to before me this____day of _____, 19_____.

IN WITNESS WHEREOF, I have set my hand and official seal:

_____
Notary Public

_____ County, _____
My commission Expires:_____

NOTARY SEAL:

Your name, address and date here

Going to:

CERTIFIED MAIL #_____

Memorandum in Law
Request for Medical Exemption Under State Statute

Dear Doctor_____:

Our particular State provides under the law a category for *medical exemption* to it's mandated vaccination policy. This exemption needs to come from a doctor of medicine, and therefore I am requesting such an exemption for _____ due to the following set of medical facts.

No vaccine can be deemed totally safe, since warnings of many symptoms and disorders arising from a vaccine can be found within the packet inserts of all vaccines the State requires by mandate. _____ could very possibly be effected adversely from these vaccines by the manufacturer's own admission, therefore _____ should receive a medical exemption.

The State of _____ has not presented me with any personal guarantee, written or otherwise, that myself or my child will NOT be harmed by said vaccines the State has mandated.

You have not presented me with any personal guarantee, written or otherwise, that myself or my child will NOT be harmed by said vaccines the State has mandated. Therefore I can safely assume that you believe some harm or risk is possible for _____, and therefore a medical exemption is warranted.

The following school officials in order (list them all), who are blocking entrance of my child to school until such vaccines are administered, have not presented me with any personal guarantee, written or otherwise, that my child will NOT be harmed by said vaccines the State has mandated. This medical exemption is necessary so that _____ can return to school.

A listing of valid research, stating that the vaccinations mandated by the State of _____ are linked to disorders such as autism, mental retardation, ADHD, decreased intelligence, cancer, disorders of the skin, allergies, disorders of the eyes and ears, sudden infant death syndrome, Parkinson's disease, dementia, Alzheimer's disease, respiratory and cardiac failure, chronic nervous system dysfunction, meningitis, encephalopathy, seizures, anemia, and epilepsy to name but a few, is included with this Request for Medial Exemption Under State Statute. Since no one can guarantee me that _____ will not receive any of these conditions as a result of being vaccinated, a medical exemption is necessary and legally indicated.

The said vaccinations mandated by the State of _____ do not guarantee that myself or my child will not acquire the diseases in which they claim to prevent, therefore a medical exemption is necessary.

There is no state of emergency regarding any of the diseases the State of _____ is attempting to control with the vaccinations mandated.

Since the majority of the population of the State of _____ is vaccinated by their own choice for themselves and their children, if it is truly the position of the State that the vaccinations mandated do control the spread of the diseases they are given for, then my choice not to vaccinate myself or my child cannot possibly create any harm to the vaccinated population.

Since the majority of the population of the State of _____ is vaccinated by their own choice for themselves and their children, if it is truly the position of the State that the vaccinations mandated do control the spread of the diseases they are given for, then my choice not to vaccinate myself or my child cannot possibly create an epidemic of any kind that poses a risk to the other citizens of the State.

The State of _____ cannot adequately prove that I am placing myself, or my child in danger of acquiring a disease by my choice to not vaccinate, since to date there have been few scientific studies on the general health of unvaccinated persons, vs. the general health of vaccinated ones, within any given population. Private research groups have studied the general health of select unvaccinated people, and the results are that unvaccinated people are generally healthier than the vaccinated population.

I am of sound mind and body, and reserve all my common law rights to non-invasion of my body, or my child's body, to chemicals being injected into us that we do not approve of, or agree with.

I am of sound mind and body, and reserve all my common law rights to make all the decisions regarding the direction of my life, and the direction of the life (lives) of my child (children), especially with regard to their safety, emotional and physical well-being.

I reserve all my rights under the *uniform commercial code,* particularly UCC 1-201, UCC 1-207 and UCC 3-501, and hereby rescind any and all contracts I may have signed with the State of _____, which caused me to unknowingly waive any of my common law rights, or rights granted to me under the constitution of the united states of America, particularly my first amendment right to religious freedom, and my ninth and tenth amendment rights to have my "*other*" rights not denied or disparaged, and protected under the common law.

I am of sound mind and body, and it is my firm philosophical belief that the said vaccinations mandated by the State of _____, have been proven by science to be extremely harmful to my body, or my child's body. Under this belief, and the belief that said mandated vaccinations will create harm to myself or my child, I hereby refuse such vaccines to be entered into my body or the body of my child without my permission and against my will. As such harm can very possibly occur to _____, a medical exemption is necessary.

I reserve all my legal rights to privacy granted to me under the Bill of Rights, the ninth and fourteenth amendments of the constitution of the united states of America. This right to privacy includes my right to control my own body, and the body of my child, and to make fundamental decisions about my life or the life of my child. Vaccines are harmful to the body, and by their very nature are an assault on the body. There is always a risk of dangerous side effects following the administration of the State of _____ mandated vaccines, as is noted by the manufacturer of said vaccines. I further declare that my right, and my child's right to privacy is fundamental at the common law, especially when the State cannot prove that my decision to not vaccinate myself or my child will in any way harm anyone, or create a potential risk to anyone. Therefore, a medical exemption is necessary for _____.

Sincerely,

STATE OF _____)
)ss
COUNTY OF _____)

BEFORE ME, the undersigned authority, _____,
known to me (or satisfactorily proven) to be the persons whose
names are subscribed to the foregoing instrument, personally
appeared and acknowledged to me that they executed the same as
their free act and deed for the purposes and considerations herein
expressed and the capacity stated, ant that the statements contained
herein are true and correct to the best of their information,
knowledge, and belief.

Subscribed and sworn to before me this_____day of _____, 19_____.

IN WITNESS WHEREOF, I have set my hand and official seal:

_____
Notary Public

_____ County, _____
My commission Expires:_____

NOTARY SEAL:

Doctors area

I, Dr. _____, licensed to practice medicine in the State of _____, hereby grant a medical exemption for _____ to not receive vaccinations for the reasons stated in this legal notice. Due to this, the medical exemption clause of our State's vaccination law applies to _____, and he/she should not receive these vaccinations mandated by the State.

Doctor's printed name _____

Doctor's signature _____

Witness _____

Witness _____

Note: to make this easier on your doctor, have him/her sign this portion in their office, and then ask for a signed confirmation of this medical exemption on the doctor's letterhead as well. Otherwise, the doctor may have to accompany you to a notary, which is unlikely. You can also have your doctor's staff cut and paste this section on their letterhead, which will save even more time.

The Church of Christ Consciousness Religious exemption to vaccinations

The church of Christ consciousness will grant you a religious exemption to vaccination. Many States will accept this as an exemption to their vaccination policies. If they do not, use the philosophies discussed in chapter 9, as well as the other forms included in this section, to help you battle the system.

The church of Christ consciousness follows doctrines that have their inception at the common law, primarily based in both versions of the Holy Bible, the teachings of Jesus, as well as other great texts and beings. When you become a member of the church, you will receive a certificate proving you are an adherent member.

The church of Christ consciousness does not require you to give up your present religion. You can be an adherent member of this church's philosophies while still practicing another family religion.

The church of Christ consciousness holds regular meetings in your home. The guidelines for such meetings are mailed to you, with a complete doctrine of the church's values and tenets. These tenets forbid the invasion of the body temple, created by God almighty, by foreign and thus man made chemicals, medications or vaccinations. The tenets do not forbid the use of medication during life threatening or crisis circumstances, and grants that the decision for these therapies are granted by God almighty to be made only by the parent of a child, or the person of sound mind and body for him or herself.

A $25 one time donation is requested for your validation of membership with the church, and to obtain the initial study materials. God bless you!

Name_____ Address _____

State _____ Zip _____ phone _____

Mail to: The Church of Universal Consciousness
34 Arcadia Road, #683
Old Greenwich, CT 06870
For further information, phone
Dr. William Trebing @ (203) 661-8122

REQUEST FOR ACCESS TO DOCUMENTS UNDER THE _____ (state) FREEDOM OF INFORMATION ACT

TO: FROM:

certified mail #
Dear (local health department or DCF official):

1. This is a request under the_____(state) Freedom Of Information Act.

2. This is a firm promise to pay fees and costs for locating, duplicating, and certifying the documents requested below. If costs are expected to exceed $50.00, please send me an estimate of the cost.

3. If some of this request is exempt from release, please send me those portions reasonably segregatable and provide me with indexing, itemization, and detailed justification concerning the information you are not releasing.

4. This information will provide knowledge and understanding of the rules and regulations of your agency, and will assist the requester relative to the policies of your agency, and the full understanding of who specifically these regulations apply to, and who specifically is authorized to enforce them.

5. I am the person making this request and my signature appears below.

6. Please send to me, the requester, copies of the *documents which demonstrate the IMPLEMENTING REGULATIONS of the state statutes, which give the authority to the Mayor*

and Health Director of (your town or city) to force me to become vaccinated, or vaccinate my children WITHOUT my consent. Please also be sure this response includes the Title, Chapter, Section and subsection or equivalent (if any), date of publication of these specific regulations, date the regulations became effective, and the page number in which they can be found on public notice in the "Regulations Of State Agencies."
Please understand that I *AM NOT* only asking for _____ General Statutes in this FOIA request, but rather, the implementing regulations as stated in the underlined portion above. In addition, please provide the IMPLEMENTING REGULATIONS of the _____ state statutes, which give the authority to the _____ Department of Children and Families to become involved in my family life upon my decision not to vaccinate.

8. Pursuant to the _____ (state) Freedom of Information Act, I am entitled to the requested documents. Please be informed that you have no legal basis for the denial of my request for non-exempt documents. I will treat the failure to comply with this request within 30 days as a final denial and pursue this matter further under the _____ (state) law. You must give me a formal receipt of this request within 4 business days.

Thanking you in advance for your cooperation.
Sincerely,

State of Connecticut　　　　　)
　　　　　　　　　　　　　　　)　　　ss.
County of Fairfield　　　　　　)

PREPARED FOR _____HOSPITAL DOCTORS,
NURSES AND STAFF
GREENWICH, CONNECTICUT

NOTICE of Patient and New Parents Rights to Refuse Medical Treatments After Childbirth
and
Release of Liability

Introductory Certification
The Undersigned, do herewith solemnly swear, declare, and state that:

We can competently state the matters set forth herewith.
We have personal knowledge of the facts stated herein.
All the facts stated herein are true, correct, and complete and not misleading, in accordance with Affiant's best firsthand personal knowledge and understanding.

Plain Statement of Facts

THE FOLLOWING NOTICED FACTS APPLY TO AS POST PARTUM MOTHER, AS FATHER OF THE NEWBORN CHILD AND THE NEWBORN CHILD

1.　Be Noticed that we are refusing all vaccinations (including hepatitis) to our newborn child and any and all INJECTIONS (including vitamin K) of any kind into the body of our newborn child. *YOU ARE NOT PERMITTED* to administer any of these medical treatments without our express written consent.

2. Be Noticed that we are refusing any treatment involving topical antibiotics applied to any part of our newborn child's body without first giving you our VERBAL consent for these treatments.

3. If a life threatening emergency occurs at any time we are at your facility for the birth of our newborn child, you MAY NOT commence medical treatments without first consulting with either of us (as new mother and as new father). We are aware that *medical vaccinations are not* used in any form of emergency care which may be necessary while we are at your facility.

4. We are aware of our rights to freedom of choice for whatever treatment we deem necessary for ourselves and our newborn child. You have no authority, and we do not recognize any authority you may assume, to demand any form of treatment or diagnostic test be imposed upon us or our newborn child.

5. We are aware of our rights to freedom within our persons and our rights to privacy granted under the common law and the constitution for these united states. You have no authority, and we do not recognize any authority you may assume, to force vaccinations, injections or antibiotics upon us or our newborn child.

6. After our child has been born, we will stay in your facility for an appropriate amount of recovery time for both mother and newborn child. At any time we feel comfortable we expect to leave your facility freely and unencumbered with our newborn child. You may not attempt in any way to detain us from freely leaving with our newborn child at any time we please.

7. Be so noticed that you have no authority, and we do not recognize any authority you may assume, to keep our newborn child at your facility without our prior express written consent. If you attempt in any way to keep our child at your facility against our will we shall consider this a criminal act of kidnapping and take appropriate action.

8. Be so noticed that you have no authority, and we do not recognize any authority you may assume, to contact or file any form of "report" with the DCF (Department of Children and Families) regarding our expression of our rights to personal freedom, and refusal of medical treatments in this matter, when have given birth to a perfectly healthy child that does not require any form of emergency care, and vaccinations are not a cure or emergency care treatment.

9. If you violate our rights to privacy in any way by contacting the DCF for our refusal to vaccinate or medicate, we will use any form you write or any words you use as evidence against any hospital personnel, and the hospital corpus in general, to commence suit for any and all damages.

10. We choose the right to freedom of choice regarding medical treatments for many personal reasons, which include both spiritual (religious) and practical. We are educated people and realize that medical treatments such as vaccinations can create long term damage to the neurological system of our newborn child, and we obviously want to avoid that at any cost, since as parents the protection of our children is our greatest priority.

11. Be so noticed that you have no authority, and we do not recognize any authority you may assume, to question us about our spiritual (religious) or practical beliefs regarding any of our above noted rights and choices. Pressing us for answers we are not willing to give you will be considered harassment and we will take appropriate action.

12. Be so noticed of these reasons we are willing to provide for choosing *NOT TO VACCINATE* our newborn child, and to *NOT* have our newborn child receive an injection of *ANY KIND* while at your facility;

    a. No vaccine can be deemed totally safe, since warnings of many symptoms and disorders arising from a vaccine can be found within the packet inserts of all vaccines the State requires by mandate.

b. The State of has not presented me with any personal guarantee, written or otherwise, that myself or my child will NOT be harmed by said vaccines the State has mandated.

c. Any doctor or nurse or hospital staff who would be administering the vaccines, has not presented me with any personal guarantee, written or otherwise, that myself or my child will NOT be harmed by said vaccines the State has mandated.

d. A listing of valid research, stating that the vaccinations mandated by the State of Connecticut are linked to disorders such as autism, mental retardation, ADHD, decreased intelligence, cancer, disorders of the skin, allergies, disorders of the eyes and ears, sudden infant death syndrome, Parkinson's disease, dementia, Alzheimer's disease, respiratory and cardiac failure, chronic nervous system dysfunction, meningitis, encephalopathy, seizures, anemia, and epilepsy to name but a few, is included with this Legal Notice.

e. The said vaccinations mandated by the State of Connecticut do not guarantee that myself or my child will not acquire the diseases in which they claim to prevent.

f. There is no state of emergency regarding any of the diseases the State of is attempting to control with the vaccinations mandated.

g. Since the majority of the population of the State of is vaccinated by their own choice for themselves and their children, if it is truly the position of the State that the vaccinations mandated do control the spread of the diseases they are given for, then my choice not to vaccinate myself or my child cannot possibly create any harm to the vaccinated population.

h. Since the majority of the population of the State of is vaccinated by their own choice for themselves and their children, if it is truly the position of the State that the vaccinations mandated do control the spread of the diseases they are given for, then my choice not to vaccinate myself or my child cannot possibly create an epidemic of any kind that poses a risk to the other citizens of the State.

i. The State of cannot adequately prove that I am placing myself, or my child in danger of acquiring a disease by my choice to not vaccinate, since to date there have been few scientific studies on the general health of unvaccinated persons, vs. the general health of vaccinated ones, within any given population. Private research groups have studied the general health of select unvaccinated people, and the results are that unvaccinated people are generally healthier than the vaccinated population.

j. We are of sound mind and body, and reserve all my common law rights to non-invasion of my body, or my child's body, to chemicals being injected into us that we do not approve of, or agree with.

k. We are of sound mind and body, and reserve all my common law rights to make all the decisions regarding the direction of my life, and the direction of the life (lives) of my child (children), especially with regard to their safety, emotional and physical well-being.

l. We reserve all our rights under the *uniform commercial code,* particularly UCC 1-201 and UCC 3-501, and Ucc 1-207 and hereby rescind any and all contracts I may have signed with the State of Connecticut, which caused me to unknowingly waive any of my common law rights, or rights granted to me under the constitution of the united states of America, particularly my first amendment right to religious freedom, and my ninth and tenth amendment rights to have my *"other"* rights not denied or disparaged, and protected under the common law.

m. We are of sound mind and body, and it is our firm philosophical belief that the said vaccinations mandated by the State of, have been proven by science to be extremely harmful to my body, or my child's body. Under this belief, and the belief that said mandated vaccinations will create harm to myself or my child, I hereby refuse such vaccines to be entered into my body or the body of my child without my permission and against my will.

n. We are of sound mind and body, and it is our firm religious belief, following the doctrine of a well organized religion, that the said vaccinations mandated by the State of, are in direct violation of my organized religious beliefs. If I am compelled to have these vaccinations injected into my body, or the body of my child, against my will, the State is violating my first amendment right to religious freedom. I have also enclosed a copy of the tenets of my religion, which prevent me and my child from receiving said vaccinations.

o. We reserve all our legal rights to privacy granted to us under the Bill of Rights, the ninth and fourteenth amendments of the constitution of the united states of America. This right to privacy includes my right to control my own body, and the body of my child, and to make fundamental decisions about my life or the life of my child. Vaccines are harmful to the body, and by their very nature are an assault on the body. There is always a risk of dangerous side effects following the administration of the State of Connecticut mandated vaccines, as is noted by the manufacturer of said vaccines. We further declare that our right, and our child's right to privacy is fundamental at the common law, especially when the State cannot prove that our decision to not vaccinate ourselves or our child will in any way harm anyone, or create a potential risk to anyone.

p. We reserve all our constitutional rights, and our rights granted to us under the common law, and herby confirm that we will prosecute the fullest extent of the law if these rights are violated in any way as a result of our decision not to vaccinate.

BE SO NOTICED THAT YOU ARE BEING RELEASED OF ANY AND ALL LIABILITY OF OUR DECISION TO NOT VACCINATE OUR NEWBORN CHILD WITH THE FOLLOWING STATEMENT:

I,(or we if two parents)_____,
hereby release you in all ways, legal and otherwise, from any liability or blame that may occur if I, or my child becomes ill to *any extent* with a disease as a result of not receiving the State of _____ mandated vaccinations.

I (or we) as a parent(s) (or human being) of sound mind and body release and totally indemnify you and your facility (hospital or otherwise) from any claim, fault, liability or blame which may occur as a result of my decision to not vaccinate myself or my child for any particular disease, whether or not such vaccines are mandated by State law. I assume full responsibility for any consequences, legal or otherwise, that follows as a result of my decision to not vaccinate myself, or my (our) newborn child.

Signed this _____ day of _____, (year) _____

Printed name _____

Signature _____

STATE OF _____)
)ss

COUNTY OF _____)

BEFORE ME, the undersigned authority, _____,
known to me (or satisfactorily proven) to be the persons whose
names are subscribed to the foregoing instrument, personally
appeared and acknowledged to me that they executed the same as
their free act and deed for the purposes and considerations herein
expressed and the capacity stated, ant that the statements contained
herein are true and correct to the best of their information,
knowledge, and belief.

Subscribed and sworn to before me this____day of ____, 19____.

IN WITNESS WHEREOF, I have set my hand and official seal:

_____
Notary Public

_____ County, _____
My commission Expires:_____

NOTARY SEAL:

Actual name of school, DCF, Health Dept, or other "official" who is giving you trouble

Address

John Henry Remedy™
In care of:
Post Office Box 9999
Los Angeles, [913XX]
California Republic

April 19, 2004

Via: U.S.P.S. Priority Mail, Delivery Confirmation # 0303 1910 0000 2097 XXXX, or certified mail, return receipt (the green thing)

Re: Citation No.: if applicable, or just school # or DCF officials badge #
Date: 03/05/04
Time Issued: 07:25 PM

NOTICE OF CONTESTED CITATION AND DEMAND FOR INVESTIGATION and CONCURRENT PUBLIC RECORDS ACT REQUEST
Pursuant to Govt. Code §§6250-6276.4

Dear _____, or Bureau dept / Disclosure Officer:

Be advised that your Oath of Office is fully accepted in all matters stated herewith.

You are hereby informed that your decision to block my child's entrance into school is contested. (In the case of an "official" trying to forcefully vaccinate your child, write: You are hereby informed that your attempt to forcefully vaccinate/medicate my child is contested. Then change

287

to body of this text accordingly). You are blocking my child from entering the school because of our family/religious decision to not be medicated by force, or without our consent. Your belief in your authority to do this is hereby Conditionally Accepted for Value, and I now as a sovereign American living soul DEMAND that you prove your authority via the PUBLIC RECORDS ACT.

Please be advised that statutory law provides fines paid to me, the requestor, of not less than $1000.00, if you do not meet the legal demands for this request.

It is hereby demanded that _____conduct an investigation in respect of the vaccination of children codes pursuant to the state of _____, and your authority to act as a representative of those codes, demonstrating proof of your delegated authority and Oath of Office to uphold the constitution of the united states.

The grounds for investigation are not limited to the following:

- No visible sign of health related difficulties in the school (be specific and state name of your particular school).
- No proof that my decision to not vaccinate my child can have any impact, or create any threat whatsoever of the general health and/or well-being of the other children or adults in the school.
- No proof that the vaccinations being demanded via_____ will add to the health of my child or family.
- No proof that the vaccinations being demanded via_____ will not further harm my child or family both physically and emotionally.
- No proof that _____ can demonstrate that the vaccination codes of the state of _____ apply to me, my children and family.
- Demandant has neither seen nor been presented with any material evidence, or likewise any material fact that

demonstrates Demandant's privacy can be violated by noted vaccination codes of the state of _____, and that these vaccination codes apply to sovereign and free Americans and their children.

This request is herby and herewith made and executed pursuant to the Public Records Act. It is further requested that the following information be provided to, without delay:

1. The legal classification that _____ (person's name), or _____ (Bureau or helath dept., whatever) is registered as in the State of _____.

2. Provide certified copies of the legal charter or articles or incorporation for (the dept in which _____ is employed by. NOTE: (This can be the department of education of your town. Most dept of ed's have no authority to dictate anything to anyone, and no legal charter. You can have a lot of fun with this!).

3. The name(s) of all executive officers or the like which are entrusted with the responsibility of managing (the depart. Of Ed, or the like. Get creative!).

4. Provide the true names of any and all public officials or private citizens employed by City of _____, (the depart. Of Ed, or the like) who are entrusted with the responsibility of Administrative Review in respect of contesting your decisions.

5. Provide the name of the administrative agency that is responsible for issuing payment to employees or officers of (the depart. Of Ed, or the like).

6. Provide the exact codes of vaccination of the state of _____you say I am in violation of, and therefore not allowed to send my child to school because of. These codes MUST be provided with the EXACT LEGAL IMPLEMENTING REGULATIONS, noted in this states Register for the public to observe, which you are attempting to apply to me.

7. Your signature under the penalties of perjury that all the above information is true and correct.

Understand that if this information is not received within 30 days I will pursue all fees allowed to me, and expect to bring my child to school. If my child is further blocked from entrance of school I will pursue the matter against you and file criminal charges with the consideration that you are a rogue agent (or organization) acting outside the confines of your delegated authority.

It is further requested that (the depart. Of Ed, or the like) waive all fees for this request. However, I am including a self-addressed, postage pre-paid envelope for your convenience.

Disclosure of the requested information to me is in the public interest, because it is likely to contribute *significantly* to public understanding of the operations and activities of City of (the depart. Of Ed, or the like), and is not *primarily* in my commercial interest.

Thank you for your consideration of this Public Records Act request.

As always, it is my pleasure to be,

John Henry RemedyÔ
Demandant

Enclosures:
Declaration (or Affidavit) of Mailing

YOU CAN NOTARIZE THIS FORM IS YOU PREFER MORE ZING

References

Law

1) Black's law dictionary—6th ed.
2) Dangers of compulsory immunizations—How to avoid them legally; T. Finn
3) Jacobson vs. Mass., 197 US 11, 25 (1905)
4) Hartman vs. May, 168 Miss 477 (1934)
5) Herbert vs. Board of Ed. 197 Ala, 617 (1916)
6) Zucht vs. king, 255 SW 267
7) Prince vs. Mass. 321 U. 158 (1944)
8) Reyes vs. Wyeth labs, 498 F 2nd 1264, 1281 (5th) Cir. Cert. Denied, 419 US 1096 (1974)
9) Davis vs. Wyeth Labs., 399 F 2nd 121, 124-5 (9th Cir. 1968)
10) Griffin vs. United States, 500 F 2nd 1059 (3rd Cir 1974)
11) Appel, Nina S., Liability in Mass Immunization Program, Bringham Young Un. Law Rev.: 1980
12) 12.42 USCA 247b (k) (2) (A) (supp. 1977)
13) Tinnerhorn vs. Park-Davis and Co., 411 F 2 d 48 (2nd Cir. 1969)
14) Polio Immunization Program, 1976 : Hearings before the Subcommittee on Health of the Senate Comm. on labor and Public Welfare, 94th congress. 2d Sess. 6 at 5-6 (1976)
15) Congressional record, Vol 83, Prt 3 (appendix & Index) p. 604, 75th congress. 2nd session
16) W. Prosser, handbook of the law of torts (4th ed.) (1976)
17) Union Pacific railway vs. Botsford, 141 US 250 at p. 251 (1891)
18) Dixon vs. US, 197 Supp 798 (WDSC 1961)
19) CSPAN; gov't reform committee Hearing on vaccines and autism, aired april 6, 2000 (information available on Cspan.com)

20) Jehovah's witness vs. King county hospital, 278 Fed. Supp. 188 (1968)

21) Whalin vs. Roe, 429 US 589 (1977)

22) Roe vs. Wade, 410 US 113 at 155 (1973)

23) Special advisory committee of oral poliomyelitis vaccine, report to the surgeon general of the public health service, at 5 (1964)

24) A history of poliomyelitis; J. Paul (1971)

25) Gottsdanker vs. Cutter laboratories, 182 Cal App. 2nd 602 (Dist. Crt. App. 1960)

26) Stahlhever vs. American cyanimid Co., 451 S.W. 2d 48 (Mo 1970)

27) Grinnell vs. Charles Pfizers Co., Inc. 274 Cal. App. 2d 424 (Dist Crt. App. 1969)

28) National Health Federation Bulletins; varying years

29) ER School of law; Michael Brown

30) Brown's lawsuit cookbook; how to sue and win; Michael Brown

31) No enforcement statutes/ IRS regulations applicable to individual income tax; Eddie Kahn

32) How to win a lawsuit without hiring a lawyer; Attny David C. Grossack

33) Cracking the Code: Third Edition.

Other Data

1. The Vaccine Reaction newsletter—National Vaccine Information Center; 1-800-909-SHOT (7468); 909shot.com

2. DPT, a shot in the dark—Barbara Loe Fisher and Harris Coulter, Ph.D.

3. Vaccination: Social violence and criminality—Harris Coulter, Ph.D.

4. DPT and chronic nervous system dysfunction—Institute of medicine, Wash DC

5. Cody CL, Baraff LJ, Cherry JD—Pertussis vaccine project: rates, nature and etiology of adverse reactions

6. Madge—The national childhood encephalopathy study

7. Griffin, M.—Risk of seizures and encephalopathy after immunization
8. Smith, R.—Where is the wisdom; the poverty of medical evidence—British Medical Journal
9. Journal of the American Medical Association archives; varying years
10. British medical journal archives; varying years
11. Lanset archives; varying years
12. Dorlands Medical Dictionary—25th ed.
13. Merck manual—13th ed
14. Guyton's Medical Physiology—6th ed.
15. Grey's Anatomy—36 ed.
16. Organic Chemistry—Streitwiesser and Heathcock 4th ed.
17. The subluxation specific, the adjustment specific—BJ Palmer, DC; vol. 28
18. The Poisoned needle—E. McBean
19. Toxemia explained—JH Tilden, MD
20. How to raise a healthy child, in spite of your doctor—R. Mendelsohn, MD
21. Confessions of a medical heretic—R. Mendelsohn, MD
22. Male practice—R. Mendelsohn, MD
23. Immunization: the reality behind the myth—Walene James
24. American natural hygiene society—varying journals
25. Marcia Dunn—Nation marks 30th year free from specter of polio—Virginian—Pilot
26. Sir William Osler—The life of Pastuer—
27. JI Rodale—Bechamp or Pasteur? Prevention magazine 1956
28. John Holt—Instead of education
29. William McGarey—The temple is beautiful—ARE press
30. Robert Olney, MD—Blocked Oxidation
31. Henry Sigerist—Civilization and disease—Cornell University press
32. The case against immunizations—Richard Moskowitz, MD
33. Alec Burton, OD—the fallacy of the germ theory of disease— talk at natural hygiene society meeting
34. AIDS Report: HIV challenged as cause of AIDS; National Times, 1992

35. The disturbing question of the Salk vaccine—prevention magazine 1959

36. The hygienic care of children; Herbert M. Shelton, ND

37. Fit for life (Vol 1 & 2); Harvey and Marilyn Diamond

38. Behold a pale horse; Wm. Cooper

39. Committee of 300; Dr. John Coleman

40. The biggest secret; David Icke

41. Roger's recovery from AIDS; Owen

42. The nontoxic home; Debra Lynn Dadd

43. Discovering homeopathy; Dana Ullman

44. The holistic pediatrician; Kathi J. Kemper, MD

45. Scientific America Magazine library archives

46. Immunization booklet; Mothering magazine

47. Don't get stuck; Hannah Allen

48. Diet for a new America; John Robbins

49. Mothering Magazine; varying issues related to vaccine induced neurological damage to children; including *"Thimerosal linked to Autism in Confidential CDC Study," March/April 2002 issue.*

50. Tedd Koren, DC: Koren Publications; *childhood vaccinations; childhood vaccination lecture materials and booklets*

51. Gary Null, Ph. D.; *Vaccines, a second opinion; 2000* with all attached references

52. I. Illich, Ph. D.; *Medical Nemesis*

53. V. Scheibner: *Vaccination, the medical assault on the immune system.*

54. H. Coulter, Ph. D.: Vaccination: Social violence and criminality

55. ***Rational Bacteriology, JR Verner, CW Weiant, RJ Watkins 1953; available @ www.soilandhealth.org***

Made in the USA
Coppell, TX
11 January 2021

47951150R20164